Mindshadows

Jean Winter

Mindshadows

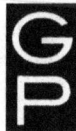

Mindshadows
ISBN 978 1 76041 156 5
Copyright © Jean Winter 2016
Cover image: Jean Winter

First published 2016 by
GINNINDERRA PRESS
PO Box 3461 Port Adelaide 5015
www.ginninderrapress.com.au

Contents

To my mother and father,
whose faith, hope and love shone
into the deepest, darkest corners of my mind,
and I knew they understood.

Introduction

This is a true account of my life, an assessment validated by factual events and logical construct. It is not just a matter of opinion, of what is right or wrong, real or imagined. The story describes my experiences in the mental health system. The diagnosis is real, the medication is real, the reports are real. While my judgement can be seen as subjective, the relevance of medical objectivity is still questionable.

Who has the power to control a person's mind and who has the answers to what is right or wrong? The medical system's attempts to do no harm have failed and the mentally ill continue to suffer.

My ideas may not be substantiated by medical authorities and it is with this in mind that I have fictionalised characters. The settings and personal names cannot be applied to any one person or institution.

The problem of categorising text as fiction or autobiography is inherent in this story, as I use a fictional character to represent 'my' reality. This novel could be seen as a fictional text trying to recreate or imagine past factualities. It has been my aim to construct a true representational autobiography. A memoir is a reflection of a life lived and therefore belongs to the author. For what is truth or reality? It is a reconstruction of ideas.

Prologue

Technological advancement in the twenty-first century has brought with it innovations, especially in medical science – improving the quality of life for those who live in developed nations. Support from private funding bodies and the government has meant that research programs can be developed. Wider education and knowledge can now be disseminated, especially with access to the world wide web.

Government economic policy and the priorities and management of resources are an ongoing issue. Major issues, especially relating to the medical and health system, always have priority. The issues surrounding a large part of society can be investigated and hopefully resolved. Unfortunately, those who are marginalised – individuals who suffer with a disability, especially a mental health condition – are not investigated with the same vivacity.

Ironically, research in this area has found that a large proportion of the population will suffer a mental illness at some time in their life. This area in the health system needs to be changed and improved. Plans for treatment and preventative measures, issues of hospitalisation, housing and support need to be understood and properly managed.

Many mistakes in diagnoses, lack of education, ignorance and fear have made detection of mental illness problematic. The medical establishment has only recently become aware of undiagnosed anxiety and depression in individuals suffering a serious illness such as cancer.

Fortunately, the health system has improved compared to past eras and areas that were under-funded are now being recognised. Those who care for the disabled or the elderly in their home are now accessing payment. Service-based consultation in the community has increased and improved the life of many people. But while there has been progress, most medical treatments in mental health have not been successful.

Conditions such as schizophrenia and other serious afflictions are not curable and can only be managed. This means recurring hospitalisation and psychological treatments can be a frustrating and sometimes a futile experience. Understanding these health conditions and improving the life of the sufferer is a multi-featured task. Medications, support networks, integration, education are necessary tools to help manage the social and practical aspects of daily life.

The ambiguous nature of mental illness creates uncertainty and fallibility in individuals who suffer the affliction. Imprisoned in another form of institutionalisation and confusing circumstances, they are defined as different, separate from the mainstream. Their attempts at integration are ruled by the indifference and fear of the wider community. They are essentially not in control of their life or destiny. Is it any wonder that those who suffer within this system feel threatened and angry with the injustice of it all?

The idea of difference is to be celebrated and not discarded. In the attempt to broaden humanity's ideals and knowledge, mental illness cannot be isolated or marginalised. Apathy and stigma will not improve understanding or society in general. Everyone needs to have self-respect and to be appreciated or recognised as important. This is not only a matter of choice, it is imperative for survival.

1

It was nine-thirty in the morning and the doctors' rooms were full. I was one of ten patients waiting my turn to be seen. The waiting room was a large hallway in a renovated bluestone villa. Two psychiatrists worked in this private practice – a Doctor Jarvie, a middle-aged woman, and her colleague, Doctor Lock, a man nearing retirement age. Their offices were located in a tree-lined street, in an affluent suburb only minutes from the city.

Doctor Jarvie was elegantly dressed in a blouse and skirt, stockings and low-heeled comfortable shoes. She looked at me and my mother, sitting waiting in the hall. I knew I was dishevelled; my long red hair was coarse and thick, my skirt and shirt stained. I knew my dark eyes were wide, sad and vacant, like I was lost in another world.

'I won't be long,' the doctor said.

I stared at the ceiling with its intricate shapes, the elegant moulding surrounding the light fixtures. I studied the printed frieze that decorated the walls. I saw the clock and watched its round face changing – a shadow forming into the image of a man. I could see his face becoming clearer. His black eyes were piercing, intense, contrasting his white face. His hair was an eruption of orange spikes. The image snarled, showing small pointed teeth. I heard a strangling, screeching voice.

You're a bitch. Why don't you inhabit other people's minds, not ours? You're just in it for the money. You're insane.

I closed my eyes and opened them again, but the vision was still there.

The abuse continued. *Your spirit's dead. The electric shock treatment didn't work — you'll rot in hell, your body will be burnt. You're going to die a cruel and violent death.*

My body was burning – flames were consuming me. My brain was being attacked. Tiny insects were jumping in my head. My body was being drained of blood. The veins and capillaries were moving my blood like water being forced through pipes. I shook my head to release the insect invasion. I wanted to scream. I looked at my mother. I made a face, baring my teeth – a demonstration of my anguish.

My mother tried to distract me from my distress. She picked up one of the magazines, flicking through the pages, showing me the glossy photos. I did not want to look at the fashionably decorated interiors, the collectible items and facades of prestigious manor homes.

I tried to understand why I was being victimised by a nasty, orange-haired devil. The only way to make sense of it was to move my head in a formation. First I pointed my head downwards, then arched my face towards the ceiling, and then I moved my head from side to side. Eventually I would look straight in front. I repeated this process several times.

My mother was looking at me.

'I'm warming up for my dance class. You know I'm the choreographer,' I said. I don't think she believed me. 'No, my head isn't going to spin all the way round.'

It was obvious to me that the reason I was seeing a doctor was because of my imminent marriage. She was going to organise my wedding to my soulmate. I would soon be walking down an aisle somewhere.

Doctor Jarvie opened the door to her room. 'Come in, please,' she said, looking at me.

I stared again at the clock. My mother took my arm.

'Yes, Mrs Baxter, you can come in too.'

My mother's tiny body moved with the help of a walker. Her back was slouched over, a dowager's hump prominent.

In the doctor's room, there were fresh roses in a china vase on the coffee table and a box of tissues. The lace curtains at the window were moving with the breeze. I could see the brilliant light. Everything sparkled. I sat next to my mother on a large cushioned sofa.

'I understand it's an emergency. What's been happening, Mrs Baxter?' the doctor said.

The doctor's desk was full of paperwork and files, layered, like the pasta sheets in lasagne. I watched as she tidied her papers, organised the prescription pads, folders, files and books. Some other paperwork – current documents, reference material related to her patients – was seemingly arrayed in a chaotic fashion. On the surface it looked disorganised, but I was sure there was a method to her madness.

Hallucinations are symptoms of deprived sleep – everyone knows that, the voice in my mind said.

My mother tried to explain the situation. 'In Felixstowe, the doctors said she had schizophrenia. But I don't believe that. I don't know what's wrong but the doctors haven't helped. They just say it's something to do with a chemical, dopamine. She wasn't hearing voices or seeing things, she was traumatised. She hasn't slept for days. My daughter isn't insane. She usually looks after herself – brushes her hair, wears clean clothes. She always takes her tablets.'

Well, I don't look too good at the moment, I thought.

The doctor kept looking through my large but condensed file and then she looked at my mother. 'She is taking her medication, I presume?' Doctor Jarvie said.

Doctor Livingstone, I presume? I thought my reaction to an old film was funny and I laughed.

'I know this is only our second appointment. My daughter has been an outpatient at Felixstowe for some time but with private hospital cover we can afford to see you. She's not very well at the moment.'

Obviously.

'The doctors wanted to change her medication all the time. She had a breakdown earlier in her life. She was twenty and she was in Felixstowe for six months. It wasn't until she came home that she got better.'

'Six months is a long time,' the doctor said.

Six, six, six, that's the devil's number.

'She didn't eat, she nearly died. The doctors couldn't do anything for her,' my mother continued.

It was all starting to make sense. I was sure I was going to be eaten.

'So what's she been like in the last few days?' said the doctor.

'She hasn't slept for three weeks now. The relaxation tapes aren't working. I thought about a hot water bottle. That helps me, when I can't sleep.'

'Where did you put that?' I said.

'So she usually lives at home with you?' said Doctor Jarvie.

'Yes.'

'What was her employment? What did she used to do?'

'She studied at university, for a degree. She's very intelligent.'

'Bachelor of chimpanzees,' I said.

'She's on a disability pension now,' continued my mother.

I knew I was saying things that were inappropriate to the conversation but they weren't listening to me. Perhaps I was invisible?

'I see. So she's been that sick?' said the doctor.

'Oh darling, don't talk to me like that. I know we've been here before, but really, dear, it is all a bit cumbersome,' I said.

I stood up because I felt like I had to arch my back and move my arms in sweeping gestures. I moved my legs, stretching them in front of me. I was a trained athlete doing a workout. I was suffering some type of cramp and trying to relieve the muscular tension.

'It must be some discomfort related to her medication,' my mother said.

I looked at my mother and knew she understood. 'I know you think I should go to hospital but you're not locking me up again, unless it's with my soulmate,' I said. 'I told the doctors at Felixstowe I was all right.'

I can't tell the truth, that there is a person living in my kneecap. If I did, the comedians would have me for lunch. I knew now that I was in fact a rat and that I was involved in some sort of expensive experiment. They were studying me, like a new species. They're going to put me in a cage and watch me go round and round on a wheel. Or will they tie me to some jumper leads and connect me to a car battery?

'Yes, go on, Mrs Baxter.'

'In hospital, she couldn't walk or talk. The nurses had to help her to the shower. She was so depressed she couldn't eat, only little bowls of custard. She was skin and bone. Now I don't think she knows what's going on, she just lies on her bed and laughs or cries.'

'I haven't slept in eighteen days,' I said. 'Wouldn't you be lost in space too? It's not my fault the sleeping tablets aren't working.' I was sure my statement was logical.

'Yes, I understand she suffers with mood swings,' said the doctor.

Mood swings! You have got to be joking. It's the medication. I wasn't going to argue, because if I did I would be sent away again.

'I know it's not right, but I don't know what to do.' My mother was trying to describe the past five years in a few sentences.

I tried not to speak. I touched my hair, running my fingers through the unruly red locks, trying to untangle the strands.

Don't tell her I'm here, okay? said a voice in my mind.

'She spent her twenty-first birthday in hospital,' my mother said. 'I know she took the drug marijuana.'

'That wouldn't necessarily be the cause of her condition – otherwise we would have a lot more people in hospital.' I knew the doctor was trying to comfort my mother. She certainly wasn't making my life easier.

Who's the patient here? Doesn't anyone want to know what I think?

'At the hospital, Gardenia couldn't stop crying and the social worker said that I shouldn't visit because I made her condition worse.'

'I understand that it must be upsetting. I also think that Gardenia was given too much medication. I've read her notes and I think the doctors misjudged your daughter. From what Gardenia says, it's the lack of sleep that's causing her distress. She may have a psychotic condition, but I do agree that the doctors at Felixstowe didn't treat her appropriately.'

Thank God someone understands.

'A man kept on molesting her, flashing his genitals – that's why they sent her to a detained area, a secure ward. They gave her that ECT.'

'Yes, electroconvulsive therapy,' said the doctor.

'But it didn't work. They're all student doctors at Felixstowe. They just treat everyone like a number.'

I looked around the room and saw the framed certificate on the wall. Doctor Jarvie was a member of the Australian and New Zealand Psychiatric Society.

'The doctors didn't ask any questions or look deeply into the matter. They just said to continue with the medication,' continued my mother. 'I would have sought different treatment for her but I couldn't afford a private psychiatrist.'

The doctor scribbled some words on her notepaper. I knew my mother was relieved. She had stopped twisting her hands in her lap.

Thank God someone is listening. It's helping her already.

'I saw my brother on the wardrobe,' I said. 'He asked me for some fruitcake.'

Do I have a brother?

I looked at the chandelier that hung from the ceiling. I could see the image of a dark shape floating. 'I'm going to have an epileptic fit. They're going to inject me with poison,' I said.

'Will she get better?' My mother looked at me and then at the doctor.

'It's a slow process, Mrs Baxter. It will take time for Gardenia to improve, but I'm sure with the right medication she will recover.'

Yeah, sure, I've heard that before.

The doctor looked at me with genuine concern. 'Do you know where you are?'

'Yes, you're Doctor Jarvie,' I said.

'That's right, but I think you should go to hospital.'

'I hate myself.' I slapped my face, repeatedly.

'Stop it, Gardenia.' My mother tried to pull my hands away.

My nose was dripping and tears were in my eyes. I could feel my brain pulsing. 'I'm not going to Felixstowe again.'

'No, you're going somewhere that's a lot nicer,' said the doctor.

'It will be okay, won't it, Mum? I don't have schizophrenia. I've never heard voices before, really. I was taking my tablets. It was the sleeping drugs that weren't working.'

'I'll give her a sedative right now, something to help her thoughts,' the doctor said. 'Then I'll take her to hospital personally. She'll be going to the

Kensington Clinic – do you know where that is, Mrs Baxter? It's on Wren Road, near Victoria Parade opposite the Fitzroy Gardens.'

'I'll find it. I'll go home and pack some clothes.'

'Yes, and can you bring Gardenia's medication, her personal details – Medicare number and health insurance numbers?'

My mother nodded.

'She needs medication, Mrs Baxter. The hospital will have a bed vacant. I'll make sure of it.' The doctor picked up the phone. She spoke to the admission staff, emphasising the urgency. 'Fortunately, they have a bed available for Gardenia. Often it's a case of waiting. Long queues are common.'

I left my mother and set out to the hospital with Doctor Jarvie. The doctor opened the door of her white BMW and I sat in the front passenger seat. We were silent as the car drove slowly through the back streets of the eastern suburbs. The clinic was only a few minutes away from the doctor's rooms.

The receptionist had arranged a taxi for my mother. I could visualise her getting into the taxi using her vouchers for a concession fare. I could see my home – a small brick maisonette – and she would be packing my suitcase with the basic necessities, pyjamas, dressing gown, day clothes, jeans and T-shirts and toiletries. I knew she would not forget my large bag of psychiatric medication.

The private psychiatric clinic was built of sandstone. It was a two-storey establishment and had an elegant appearance. I noticed the purple-flowered bougainvillea vine crawling around the front pillars. The delicate small pansies near the door did not assuage my apprehension.

The doctor and I walked through the main foyer. In the reception area I saw the rich furnishings – upholstered armchairs, a large oriental vase with long stems of purple and white irises standing on a polished hallway table.

I was led into a small room. We were soon joined by a nurse in a blue uniform.

'This is Gardenia Baxter,' Doctor Jarvie said to the nurse. 'She'll be here for a little while. Her mother will be arriving shortly and she'll help with the admission details. Can you take Gardenia to her bedroom and give her some medication, risperdal? She's displaying psychotic symptoms. She's cognisant to know where she is, but I'd like you to check on her continually. I'll come in later and take care of the admission notes and write up her current medication. Okay?'

The nurse nodded.

I watched Doctor Jarvie walk out of the clinic. I looked at the nurse, who had a name badge on. I read the word 'Julia'.

'I'll take you to your room. It looks out onto the garden.' The nurse led me through a warren of hallways and passages.

We came to a room which had a sign next to the door, number twenty-three. I entered a sunlit room.

'There are some forms to fill in, but you can do that later,' Julia said.

I looked at the oak desk and the white and blue brochures.

'One is for the menu, and you need to take that to the dining room. Afterwards I have to take your blood pressure, okay?'

She's like a bird, pick, pick, pick.

'I'm just depressed, I don't need to be here really,' I said. I didn't want to say that I was going mad.

'Having a mental illness is difficult,' said Julia.

Is she being patronising? I'm not an idiot.

'It's lunchtime now, so I'll get you a sandwich and a drink. I'll leave you to settle in.' Julia left the room.

Settle in?

Great to be back. The voice in my mind had returned. It's nice here. Can't we stay forever? It's much better than Felixstowe, isn't it?

It's just my unconscious mind, made audible. It will go away. My God, I haven't been sleeping, that's all. I've been battling to have power over my own mind, to make my own conclusions. I feel like an out-of-date product, a piece of meat, like a pie, that's sitting in the frozen meat section of the grocery store. They're not going to eat me, are they?

I looked around the room. It consisted of a bed, desk and wardrobe. I saw a red button placed near the door, saying 'Emergency'. A jug of water and a glass were on the desk, with a small vase of flowers. Clean fluffy white towels sat on the floral bed cover. Another door led to a bathroom. I went into the room and looked at my reflection in the mirror. Long strands of string hung from my head. My eyes were large and black. I looked like a strange and exotic type of animal, a monkey.

I stared at the bathroom tiles and saw blood drip down from the ceiling; everything was red. I looked at the shower cubicle and I could see myself standing naked, my body cut and bleeding. I looked away.

I tried to form an idea – to logically assess the horror I was seeing and feeling. I sat on the bed; my fear was crippling. In my mind, images of black squares were floating and patterns of plus and minus symbols used in mathematics were jostling for attention. I tried to push them into the corner of my mind. I heard a voice.

I know the answer to the meaning of life. It's in the bathroom.

I quickly ran out of the room and found my way back to the main reception area. I saw my mother sitting, waiting with my suitcase by her side.

'Can I help you?' Julia, the nurse, was speaking to my mother.

'Yes, I'm Mrs Baxter. My daughter has just been admitted.' My mother saw me as I ran down the passageway.

'Here I am, Mum. I'm okay, just keeping up with my exercise plan.'

Did they really want to know what I had just seen in the bathroom? Not a nice topic of conversation, but then I was in a mental hospital.

'We have to fill in some admission details. Will you both come with me?' The nurse picked up the suitcase and my mother pushed her walker.

We followed the nurse into another small room. The consulting rooms were positioned on either side of the hallway. The small room consisted of a desk and chair for the doctor or staff and a two-seater sofa decorated in a floral chintz pattern.

'We just need details.' Julia directed us towards the sofa.

I was able to answer the questions, my general practitioner's name, my address, date of birth. My mother had my health care cards and the numbers were recorded. I watched as the nurse placed stickers on various pieces of paper.

'I need a drink of something,' I said.

'Of course. I'm nearly finished.'

We waited and when the nurse had tidied her papers, we left the room. That was the first time my mother had participated in the admission process and by her smile I could see she was pleased.

'Can I see Gardenia's room?' she said.

'Of course, just follow me,' said Nurse Julia.

The nurse took my suitcase and we walked towards the southern end of the hospital. We took a different route and we passed a large room, with comfortable armchairs surrounding a coffee table. I saw three red phones placed on the wall, large boxes with a receiver and slots where coins could be inserted. A large fish aquarium was in the corner. I saw tropical fish, dazzling in their colour and decoration, swimming in the container. An ornate fireplace with a container of brass pokers was situated on the opposite wall. I was surprised that they allowed such tools in a hospital like this.

We came to my room – number twenty-three.

Julia smiled as she placed the suitcase near the door. 'If you have any questions or need help, just come and see us at reception, okay?'

I nodded.

'Thank you,' said my mother. 'They're very nice here, don't you think so, Gardenia?'

A hospital isn't a nice place. I don't care if they are nice or not. It's certainly better than a public hospital. I'll agree with that. Although who knows what's going to happen next?

My mother sat down on the seat next to the desk. I poured myself a glass of water and then offered my mother a drink. I sat down on the bed and looked out of the window.

'It's a lovely place, clean, beautiful things everywhere. You have your own bathroom, very luxurious.'

'Yes, I even get room service.' I knew my mother was putting on a brave face. 'She's a good doctor, everything will turn out fine – I'm a lucky girl.'

No it won't. I'm a bloody loony. Why do I have to excuse myself and understand my mother's distress? Everything is not all right and I am not happy to be here. I felt guilty for not appreciating my mother's help. *It's not her fault, but she did leave me at Felixstowe. I'm dependent on her, but can I trust her? I'm terrified of society but I have no one else to lean on for support. The Felixstowe doctors think she's a rational woman and they have to agree with her wishes.*

We sat in silence for some time.

'It's like a first-class hotel, isn't it? I feel like a film star, on a health farm.' I felt like I was acting. 'I could win an academy award for this. Thank you, ladies and gentlemen, the foreign press, my colleagues, you have all been like a family to me. I don't think I deserve this award, but then I have been through hell to get it.'

Perhaps it is just like being an actor – losing yourself, your identity, to become another person. Will the real Gardenia Baxter please stand up?

The nurse Julia returned. 'Gardenia, your doctor's here and I have a tablet to give you. It'll help,' she said.

I took the tablet, hoping it would make me sleep. I felt like I was jumping in the sky from one cloud to another. I was trying very hard not to slip off the vaporous white pillows. Everything was farcical, contradictory. I knew I could fall through the clouds because they weren't solid matter but I hoped for stability none the less. My mind was like a milkshake being pummelled by a mechanical masher. I wondered if the psychiatric hospitals were the cloud formations and the doctors were the mixing beaters and I was the milkshake. I thought my metaphor was strikingly accurate.

I'll have to write that down.

My mother and I followed Julia to the reception area and sat in the hallway, near the consulting rooms.

'Just wait here and the doctor will be with you shortly,' Julia said.

My mother and I sat on the blue padded armchairs. I noticed that everything was blue, most of the soft furnishings, the upholstery and cushions. The walls were a pale orange colour. The complementary colour scheme didn't improve my despair. A teasing voice spoke in my mind.

Do you think she can help you?

Doctor Jarvie walked down the hallway. 'Come in, Gardenia. Mrs Baxter, will you join us too?'

I sat on another plush comfortable chair. My mother pushed her walker and sat down next to me.

I'm someone special and I'm in an important meeting. I'm a consultant. The doctor's asking for my advice on relevant mental health issues. She'll learn from my experience.

'So why do you think you're here?' Doctor Jarvie was looking at me but I wondered why she was asking me such a question.

She's the doctor. Can't she answer that? Oh, I was just in the vicinity and decided to admit myself just on the off chance of getting a meal. I don't think she'd like to hear my sarcasm.

'How are your thoughts now?'

Oh God, do I have to go through all this again?

'I guess I'm sick.' *I can't say I'm well. I want to trust the doctor and the nurses.* I could see that they were being kind, but did they have ulterior motives? 'I'm tired, frightened.'

'The new medication will help. What are you frightened of?' the doctor asked.

'The hospital.'

'Why?'

'I don't know. I think I'm depressed.'

'Have you had thoughts of suicide?'

'Yes, no, I'm okay.' I didn't want to say that my mind wasn't working properly, although that was obvious to everyone. To admit it meant the likelihood of institutionalisation. I didn't want to be locked up again.

What is the reason for my illness? Manic depression – high and low mood swings. Is it schizophrenia and what does that mean? Is medication the only remedy? A hospital is a place where sick people get better, don't they? I had asked these questions so many times and I still remained confused. *Does Doctor Jarvie have any idea?*

'I do have Gardenia's notes from Felixstowe – her past psychiatric history. Obviously her condition has not improved and the medication is not working. I understand that various medications will have to be considered and observation with continual reassessment is the only viable option. Even so, I do need to hear your opinion, Mrs Baxter.'

'I know she was on lithium and I think haloperidol,' said my mother.

She was my saviour now. I couldn't think, remember, or even qualify as being human.

'Do you think the medication is working, Gardenia?'

'No.'

'They had her on tegretol, is that the right name?' said my mother.

'Why did they put Gardenia on tegretol, Mrs Baxter?'

'She had an epileptic fit, but I think that was due to another medication. I think they found a lesion in her brain. Doesn't it stop muscular spasms? I don't really know.'

'I see. It can also help a mood disorder,' said Doctor Jarvie. 'You're still taking the major tranquillisers. How are they affecting you, Gardenia?'

I looked at her blankly. I wondered what world she was on, perhaps Neptune. *Can I give a reply – does she think the tablets are working? Perhaps she just wants to know how I'm feeling, what's going on?* 'I can't concentrate or think logically, if that makes sense.'

'It makes perfect sense. I'll put you on a new medication, something that is not from the dark ages. Tegretol has too many side effects anyway.'

'I did get better after leaving Felixstowe,' I said.

If she's going to change my medication, even lessen it perhaps, then that's not so bad. She actually thinks I have a brain. Well, it's her job to realise I have a brain. She's actually asking for my opinion and she's taking me seriously.

'I'll keep you on an antipsychotic but something a bit less corrosive.'

'I think I've already rusted.'

The doctor laughed. 'Don't worry. I'll fix you up, even if we have to use some anti-rust. What else are you feeling, Gardenia?'

'I'm depressed that I can't do things like I used to. I did go back to study but I feel like I've lost my personality.'

I could not give an answer or a clear definition of what was wrong. I was angry with my previous treatment and although I thought they had misjudged me, I was uncertain of my own sanity – I was not coping. I had never been floridly psychotic like this before.

'We'll get you well first and then we can think of a career for you.'

I stared at the doctor in disbelief.

'Are you on any antidepressants, Gardenia?'

'No, I think I was on them for a short period but they took me off them.'

'They can help with anxiety too,' said Doctor Jarvie. 'I'll start them tomorrow. I also think the alprazolam three times a day will help ease the anxiety. It is a minor tranquilliser and it is an addictive medication, but as a short-term solution is very useful. Also, I don't think you have an addictive personality.'

'Do you think the doctors at Felixstowe gave Gardenia the wrong medication?'

My mother wanted the truth, I could tell.

'Perhaps as a public institution they're under-funded and therefore evaluations can be a hurried affair. Sometimes the consequences are more harmful than the original complaint.'

'Yes, I think it will all help,' I said. 'I'll just take your tablets now and I'll go home. Great, well, thanks very much.' I stood up to leave.

'Gardenia, you're going to stay in hospital for a little while. How do you like this place? It's not so bad, is it?' Doctor Jarvie had very good marketing skills.

'It's different – I mean, from Felixstowe. I don't want to blame the medical system, but it was a frightening place. Can trauma make you psychotic?' I was going to leave if I could just make the doctor see that I was all right, that there was a reason for my sickness. Then I could just go home.

'Yes, certain kinds of shock can have a marked effect and I agree Felixstowe could be improved. I fully understand your anxieties. On behalf of the mental health system, I would like to apologise.'

I was trying hard to take this explanation seriously.

'I feel like I've lost something. Have I had some sort of amnesia?' I was beginning to feel less threatened. I could tell that the doctor was listening, trying to understand. *Will she condemn or judge me, tell me I'm insane?*

The doctor was writing down notes. It was a usual occurrence for me to see this. I had never asked what it was they were writing – perhaps I was too afraid to hear the response. They never voluntarily disclosed their ideas. I knew Doctor Jarvie was writing down a report that was not for my eyes.

'Every time I reach for something to hold onto, it disappears. I want to focus on what you've just said and why, but as soon as I do, I forget the reason why I was trying to focus on it in the first place.' I looked out the window and saw the curling flowers of the grevillea. I was pretending it was a normal thing to do, to appreciate beauty. I was avoiding eye contact. 'It's hard if your thoughts aren't connected. To make any decisions, make an argument or resolve issues. I feel like I'm a blank space. A person walking but dead inside. It's confusing. The voices or hallucinations I haven't had before, not like this. I'm sure it has something to do with not sleeping.' I moved my hands, thinking I was communicating with an elaborate system of sign language. I could see the doctor looking at my hand gestures. I stopped waving my arms in the air. *She thinks it's a sign of my insanity.*

'I don't want to have this illness and even if I have an illness, what's the reason?' I said. 'It must be more than a chemical dysfunction. I wish life could be that easy.'

'Have you ever been to classes, dealing with problem solving and CBT?' said Doctor Jarvie.

I shook my head.

'We have very good programs, which I think will be beneficial. I'll write down an outpatient program for you. It's covered by your health insurance.'

'What's CBT?' *It sounds like some kind of sexually transmitted disease.*

'Cognitive behavioural therapy. It helps to restructure your mind, to be aware of your thoughts and how they affect your feelings. Behavioural change can be implemented.'

I didn't understand it, but it sounded good. My thoughts turned to mice in cages and then I remembered my own rabbits at home. Did they have enough water? Could Mum look after Bessie, my border collie?

'The antidepressant will take four or five days to take effect. I'll see you tomorrow night and we'll talk more about it, okay? I think having a good sleep tonight will make you feel better.'

I agreed with her last statement – that's if I could sleep. I had visions of myself gradually dying staring into space, unable to close my mind. I had never experienced such unrelenting pain before. I was a vegetable that momentarily had sparks of illumination, confirming my identity as an edible plant.

Can antidepressants help potatoes? Can the doctor differentiate between different species of potatoes? I don't look like a potato, do I?

'I need the sun,' I said. 'With warmth, good soil, better surroundings to grow in and lead a productive life.'

'Yes, she does need to build her body up,' my mother said.

'You are my watering can, my blood and bone. I can't swim. I will just fall to the ground like a ripened potato.' My attempt to appreciate their help was ignored.

'I think changing the medication will help.' The doctor looked at my mother. 'I think Gardenia has needed antidepressants for some time and her anxieties need to be addressed. It's probable they didn't place her on the antidepressants because they thought it would exacerbate the psychosis or elevate her mood. But the first thing to do is to quieten her thoughts.'

My mother nodded.

'I think in two weeks' time, she'll be able to leave the hospital. I've made some notes in relation to an outpatient program, which I think will be very helpful. I don't think she'll have any more episodes. With continual reassessment, I think her problems can be solved. Do you have any questions, Mrs Baxter?'

I looked at the doctor. Her eyes were watery and I wondered if she was crying.

'I'm getting older and I want Gardenia to be independent. I want her to have a happy life.'

'I fully understand. When we have the medication right, we can look into rehabilitation services and in this way, I think Gardenia will improve.'

'Did her brain shut down like eyes do, to block out the sunlight? Has Gardenia's life been too hard? Has her brain stopped working, so it can rest, so it can still function? Is that why people call it a "nervous breakdown"?'

I thought my mother was very intelligent to use a metaphor like that. I knew she understood my wish to live in a glasshouse.

'The brain can shut down in a way, which enables it to survive. I imagine that it's a part of our system, to find alternate ways to operate. I am not sure in Gardenia's case that she has a physical aberration, in terms of a dysfunction. I think psychological treatment would be more appropriate. It's also a good idea to look for the cause of Gardenia's illness too.'

'What do you think about that?' My mother looked at me as if all my problems were over.

I didn't want to disappoint her. 'I think it sounds all very good.'

'Okay, that's settled. Thank you, Mrs Baxter, and Gardenia, I'll see you tomorrow night, okay?'

We left the doctor and walked to the large lounge area where the tropical fish lived.

'Though the way is long, let your heart be strong keep right on to the end.' My mother could not sing in tune but it didn't matter. She was by my side and that was the most important thing. Her courage and sincerity was my lifeline. 'I think that's the best thing that has happened to us in a long time, Gardenia.'

'I'll be home soon, won't I, Mum, and they won't keep me here? I'll get stronger and I'll be able to help more.'

I visualised my home. I had planted garden beds at the front and side. I had designed a cottage garden with an arch and climbing roses. I knew the succulents and native trees and bushes would survive, especially in this dry summer heat, but would the roses die?

'I don't feel as stressed and I think the change in the medication will help.' I felt tired and I didn't want to talk. I wasn't going to ask my mother to water the roses; she had enough to do. Obviously I was a nuisance and she couldn't look after me any more.

I do look after myself. I haven't been able to sleep, that's why I'm unwell. I wanted to believe everything would be all right. To tell my mother I felt better. I had to keep on going, both metaphorically and physically.

I had tried so often to get back on track. Unfortunatel,y the train I waited for never came along. Maybe it was now time to find myself transport, to make the journey with the help of a good navigator? Doctor Jarvie seemed to know where she was going.

My mother wanted to go home. She looked tired. She had not been sleeping well, worried about my health. I had been wandering around the house at night, often talking out loud and having conversations with the characters in my mind. It had been okay for a while having humorous discussions with television personalities and comedians. It had only been in the last few days that the voices had turned sour.

I walked with my mother to the front entrance. I waited with her until the taxi arrived.

'Remember, Gardenia, there are more sick people outside of institutions than inside them.' A profound saying, but I understood her. 'You must always believe in yourself.'

I nodded. It was easier said than done.

'Chickens always come home to roost, Gardenia, and you'll come home too.'

That proverb was a mystery to me. Should I cackle? But then this was serious. I was in a mental hospital and pretending to be a chicken was not a good idea. Mind you, I had just told the doctor I was having an identity crisis, thinking of myself as a potato. It couldn't get any worse, could it?

'Can we afford this?' I said. 'Only the rich can afford to go to health retreats, private hospitals.'

'Mental disorders cross all economic boundaries but the intensity of the suffering is the same for both rich and poor. Money does help, but can't cure some disorders,' my mother said.

I didn't want to try and understand, especially theories of capitalism and the mental health system. I couldn't help myself from participating in an intellectual debate.

'Well, that's positive thinking. It helps the pharmaceutical companies and the health insurers and the government – they make money,' I said. I wanted to change the subject to talk about my health and my circumstances. 'Will I get better, Mum? I won't always be in mental hospitals, will I?' I knew such a question couldn't be answered. I was looking for encouragement and I did wonder what she was going to say next or what I was going to think or hear or do.

'Schizophrenia's only a label, Gardenia, but each individual's different. It's necessary to have a name for a condition. There are various types of cancer and some are not as serious as others.'

She's being very sensible, isn't she? a voice in my mind said.

'Some people are like ponies and some like racehorses. If you're a pony, you can't carry a load like a draught horse and you shouldn't be expected to.'

I wondered if I was a pony.

'People with imaginative minds are either blessed or cursed. They know greater fear because they can imagine it. You can create, Gardenia, and you should be very proud of yourself.' My mother smiled. 'You'll be all right,' she said.

Proud of myself being a loony, that I talk to devils, take a bucket load of medication and really don't have a bloody clue what's going on? Plus my mother thinks she's Jesus Christ talking in parables. I think I'm doing well not to murder everyone right now and tell them what idiots they are.

'There's nothing wrong with me, Mum. I'm just depressed. I'll be home soon.' I was now wondering if I wanted to go home.

'An end is just another beginning, Gardenia. You won't suffer like this again.'

A voice in my mind spoke and I was sure it was Jesus Christ. *I think she's talking about Genesis. It is written.*

'Well, if it's written, then why are you talking to me about it?' I said back to the son of man.

You should listen to her. She makes a lot of sense, said Jesus.

Well, I can't help it, can I? I felt like telling Jesus to clear off and then thought better of it.

'I'll be back tomorrow,' my mother said.

I laughed out loud. *This is hysterical. I'm in a mental home having an argument with Jesus. Just as well I have a sense of humour.*

'I'm glad you're feeling better. It's good to hear you laugh, Gardenia.'

I've been carrying on like this for the last three weeks. What's so different? Maybe it's because I'm in hospital and she thinks things are looking up.

I did want to go with her, even if I was getting frustrated with her wise words, but the thought of listening to Jesus Christ all day wasn't appealing.

A man dressed in blue pants and a white shirt came into the foyer. He was obviously the taxi driver. The emblem on his shirt proved it. I watched my mother slowly rise from her chair.

She gripped my arm and gave me a big smile. 'It won't be for long, Gardenia.'

I watched her move the walker in the direction of the door. I didn't want to think about how much I loved her. I didn't want to add to my suffering.

I went back to my room to unpack my clothes. I still couldn't get over the luxurious surroundings. I felt like I was in a first-class hotel but this fantasy didn't last long as I noticed that the hangers in the wardrobe were fixed.

Although they do that in hotels, don't they? I wondered if the other patients would steal my belongings. *Mind you, I don't have designer clothes or a diamond necklace.* I felt like I was playing a role in a real-life documentary, a satire on mental illness. *Perhaps I could be a film director?* If only I had a control console to direct the mechanisms of my mind. I could at least know the outcome. I'd have a happy ending.

I was in the dark, not literally, but suddenly I did feel a sense of hope, like daylight penetrating through a crack in a door.

It's the fog of fear, the voice said. I was sure it was Jesus Christ again.

'Change is frightening, Jesus,' I said.

Most things are, he replied.

'I don't want to go in the bathroom.' I wanted his reassurance.

I don't blame you.

Well, at least he knows how I'm feeling. If anyone can sort this business, he should be able to. Perhaps I'm really on stage, involved in a theatre production. The voices and my thoughts are a fantasy, a fiction being enacted but without the stage direction. I'm just suffering symptoms of trauma, exacerbated by the conditions in the public system. Six months in an institution, in continual fear and not in control of your life, would make most people terrified.

Night didn't come soon enough. I had another sandwich for tea. They didn't mind me staying in the bedroom. I took the medication and then put on my pyjamas. I washed my face and brushed my teeth. I wasn't scared of the bathroom, knowing that Jesus was with me. I pulled back the clean crisp sheets and lay down. I wondered if I should lock the door. I could hear screaming and noise from outside, people shouting. I wondered if it was real, but remembered that I was not in Felixstowe.

Gradually my tension subsided. The strong medication was making an impact and slowly the noise lessened. The cries were diminishing, until everything was silent. It was the first time I had felt peace in a long time. I had fallen asleep.

I dreamt of a butterfly emerging from a chrysalis. I saw an ugly duckling growing and turning into a swan. I saw my home and my mother welcoming me with open arms.

2

I was lying on the hospital bed. There was just enough light to make out the furniture – the chair, desk, chintz curtains and a watercolour landscape print on the wall. I wondered where I was and tried to recollect the past.

Then I heard the voices again.

You are my dream lover, the person I have always longed for.

I suddenly felt a strong connection to something that was good. It assuaged my fear and I felt liberated, a sense of freedom.

Then another voice spoke. You have an important purpose and you are not having a near – death experience and no, you won't go to heaven.

Then many voices spoke in my mind. They started to argue.

I'm talking to her. No, I'm talking to her. I saw her first.

Shut up all of you. Don't you understand I'm in a hospital because of you lot. Can't you understand my predicament? I wondered if talking logic could persuade them to leave my mind.

I looked towards the door, hoping no one could hear my conversation.

I'm talking in my mind. They can't hear that, can they? I'm not paranoid, but talking to people who aren't there is not a 'normal' thing to do.

'Who are you?' I said to the voices, hoping if I could understand their reasons for pestering me, I could find out how to get rid of them.

I'm a star, said a voice.

Who are you really? You must be someone, I said to the voice.

Don't you know? I'm the one who has always loved you. I wasn't sure if such a thing was possible.

Oh, go on. You don't really love me that much. Do you? You're not a film star, are you? .

No, but I am good-looking, charming and so in love with you, it's overwhelming.

32

I was overwhelmed too. I felt like a teenager flirting with my first boyfriend.

I'm all of your favourites. I'm stars wrapped in to one, the voice said.

Yeah, in your dreams, said another voice.

Do you have loads of money? I said to the mystery person in my head. I wondered if I could make this illogical thought process practical.

Now why would you want that? Love isn't about money, is it?

It certainly helps. You can't go very far without it, you know, I replied. I was tired of this constant intense conversation. Talking inside my head was exhausting.

I'm not telling you my name, because you're only after me for my money. The voice was angry.

Oh God, all my dreams have come true. You do have money!

I wondered if the voices were my 'inner child'. *People listen to this type of thing, don't they? I love you,* I thought, hoping I could take over the conversation. *I'm important and I can see the world again. I can see me, as before. Not as I am now. My prison is quiet and I need to understand that people are meandering, not going anywhere. I will see you, my inner child, for you are in me and I am in you. The world is seen through a thousand eyes. The past has gone and the future is not here. Only the present remains when I see you.*

I was sure affirmations had their place in overcoming negative thinking. I knew that the voices were my own thoughts. I was trying to discover my real purpose on this earth. I felt sure that if I convinced my mind of this, then everything would be okay.

What a load of rubbish. Are you being serious?

I was sure my inner child was trying to be prophetic.

This philosophy stuff, doesn't it make you confused?

Well, if you don't want to talk to me, you don't have to.

I do not want to talk to you any more. Goodbye. Anyway, your teacher will come when you're ready, said the voice.

Good, that got rid of him.

Suddenly there was a knock on the door. A young nurse came in. She looked happy and I wondered why.

'Good morning, Gardenia. It's eight o'clock and breakfast is ready in the dining room. I'm your nurse for today, my name is Celia.' She was short and had a voice that squealed.

I remembered the mice, in my childhood, when my father used to feed them poison. They didn't die straight away. I was able to pick them up, because they were too sick to move quickly. I thought if I could put them up in the roof of the garage, they'd get better. I'd be able to free them from my father's genocidal tendencies.

'Did you sleep well?'

'Yes, I just woke up from a dream. It was about mice,' I said.

'Oh, that's nice. Good dream, was it?' Celia looked interested.

'Mice are strange creatures, aren't they?'

'Yes, sometimes,' Celia said.

She doesn't know how to answer that question. I suppose we're all strange.

'I'm in hospital, aren't I?'

'You were admitted yesterday. You're in Kensington Clinic. Don't forget after breakfast you have to take your medication, okay?'

Celia was standing by the door looking at me with eyes that had dark shadows underneath. I wondered if she needed vitamins.

Why do they always go on about medication? Don't they have something else to think about? Can't they occupy their day by doing something useful?

Celia was still standing by the door staring at me.

At least she makes personal contact. She did call me by my name and she smiled. Then she is paid, but the nurses and doctors were given a wage at Felixstowe. It made a change for someone to talk to me in a nice manner. I felt like I was on a holiday. I felt better already. She had white bright teeth. I thought she could be in advertising, proclaiming the importance of good dental routine.

'You've missed your calling, Celia.'

'Really? Why is that?'

'Because you look like a model,' I said.

Am I grovelling, because she couldn't go on television with a hooked nose, could she?

You're a bitch. The voice had returned.

I tried to ignore the remark, thinking it was my fault for seeing Celia as ugly.

'Oh, don't be silly,' she said. Celia giggled like a little girl.

'You want to be known for your intelligence,' I said. I thought I was getting better with small chit-chat.

'Come with me, Gardenia, and I'll show you the dining room.'

I saw myself as a successful entrepreneur. Celia was my secretary and this five-star hotel suite was part of the job's requirements. I was here for a business meeting. I had engineered the process. It was a better alternative than thinking I was sick in the mind.

I was pleasantly surprised to find my dressing gown and slippers in the wardrobe.

I followed Celia down the passage way. I noticed the art prints on the wall – European masters, like Cézanne and Van Gogh. I looked at another print – an Australian impressionist painting by Fred McCubbin. A scene showing a little girl lost. It made me feel homesick.

The large dining room consisted of small booths, tables, a serving area and a long counter where patients ordered and selected their meals. Tea, coffee, cereals and milk were provided. People were already sitting, eating. They looked as though they had been violated, woken far too early. As if it was a hard task to participate in any morning ritual, even to eat a meal already cooked and prepared. I thought that the patients' behaviour was understandable. After all, it was a hospital and it was acceptable and 'normal' to feel lousy.

I joined a small queue and asked for a small tub of yogurt. I felt like an outsider, sitting alone at the back of the dining room nearest the exit door. Not many of the patients sat together. There were only a few who did like company. Those patients who delved into their problems, finding solace with others who were in similar dilemmas. I wondered if they came into hospital to enjoy comforts they could not get elsewhere. I questioned their motives.

Why would they suffer, go through hell, just to have some physical luxury? It's not a healthy way to go through life. If they like hospital, having meals prepared and comfortable beds, then obviously they are sick in the mind. Who wants to be in hospital? If the patients found life difficult at home, stressed by their incapacity to deal with issues, they certainly would not be alone. If that is the case, they aren't really sick at all. More likely they're very intelligent and know how to work the system.

I understood that hospital would be a preferred option. I could not question their rationality in wanting to sleep in beds with clean sheets and have a roast dinner on a Sunday. Who wants to lie in the gutter in rags talking to an electric light pole? The hospital had wonderful amenities but it was still a depressing and morbid place.

If I need a rest, I should go on a holiday. Isn't that a more 'normal' reaction? I forgot long ago how to have fun or be social. Why am I in this hospital?

I listened to the nursing and dining staff talking, exchanging pleasantries. I heard them comment on cooking rosters, patients' medication, what they did on the weekend. I remembered the past, images of the dining area at Felixstowe. I could see four young men, tormenting an older woman. She was sitting at the back, quiet and withdrawn, her hands shaking as she tried with great effort to put food in her mouth.

'Hey, Cindy, have you wet your pants today?' One of the men said and the offensive group laughed. 'Is it time to put your nappies on? Then you couldn't put them on yourself? Would you like me to help you?' The group laughed again. 'Only you have to pay me.'

I remembered the woman screaming and her body writhing in convulsions. I didn't see her again, but I did see the men. It was likely that Cindy was taken to a secure ward, but she had not offended or violated or committed a crime. I was sure the men were not punished or reprimanded. I could not forget my experiences in Felixstowe. The public hospital was like an abattoir. Like a stuffy caged prison, and the patients were like cattle, observed without hope of escape. I could still hear the hysterical pleas of inmates and see the patients' staring eyes. They were lost, sad individuals, without hope. It was not a place where recovery was possible. It was a place of terrifying proportions, a gaol sentence many serve, without having committed a crime.

Can a person without an illness live in such an environment and not be psychologically affected for the rest of their lives? Is it any wonder the community fear such places?

The memory was put on hold when I heard the sound of another voice.

'I've been looking for you,' Celia said.

I wanted to say the obvious, that I was still in the hospital, had not run away or committed any heinous offence, or taken my own life or another's. I refrained from complicating the conversation.

'How are you settling in? It's always difficult the first night.'

'Oh yes, I think so.' I felt like I was stepping on quicksand and the soft liquid was oozing around me. If I made the wrong move, I would certainly feel the repercussions. 'I did notice a nurse with a torch shining a light on me a few times.' They did that too at Felixstowe, but I was getting accustomed to their methods.

'I have some medication for you at the nurses' station. After you finish breakfast, we'll catch up, okay?'

'I'll try.'

I wondered how we were going to catch up. *Who's going to be caught? Will I find her passing down a corridor? Will I chase a white rabbit down a hole?* The hospital was like a warren with its passageways. I was worried that I didn't have the answer.

After breakfast, I went to the nurses' station to take my medication. I logically assumed it was the best way of contacting the staff. I knew they weren't rabbits. I passed the red phones in the large room and remembered the many times I rang my mother from Felixstowe, asking to be taken home. I saw the fish swim in the large aquarium.

Just as well they don't have a memory. Talk about futility. I felt like a lost soul swimming in a fish bowl. I hated taking the tablets, having to throw my head back, nearly choking. I didn't like the idea of having a drug altering my thoughts. *But if they can work and make me feel better, then there is some benefit.*

The nurses' station looked an uncomfortable place. It was a small room, with glass panes. There was a small opening between the window and the desk. It was similar to an old-fashioned banking system where a protective screen shielded the teller from the client. The small space allowed for the transference of money. I knew this aperture was used for dispensing tablets to patients. I sat down on a nearby chair and watched and waited.

A nurse was busy in the room. She reminded me of a sparrow, picking at crumbs with her fingers. She made jerky movements as she moved around the room. She looked about sixty years of age. I hoped she wouldn't fall off her perch. I knew it was not a nice simile and felt guilty because of it.

More nurses started to arrive, until there was not much room left in the glass cubicle. They were trying to engage in some appropriate manner of moving, pushing past each other, explaining the reason for their existence. I watched an old man in a suit try to get in, vying for space. He was certainly the top pigeon, probably the doctor, because the nurses moved out of his way. He wasn't wearing a uniform, so that substantiated my theory. The staff reminded me of fish captured behind glass; the nurses were the small goldfish and the doctor was the big groper. Most of their duties were a mystery to me. I knew the files were kept in alphabetical order and the reason why the cabinets and doors were locked.

Would a patient want to steal their own medication? I could imagine it being a possibility: 'Excuse me, but you haven't given me enough antipsychotic. I want to be sedated so I can't even walk.' Who knows? After all, we were mentally ill. I saw a vision of a child in a Charles Dickens novel saying, 'More please. I don't want potatoes but I would like the green tablets, thank you.'

I watched as the staff one by one left the office, the last nurse locking the door behind her. I sat and waited for Celia.

Every now and then, I would see patients in their dressing gowns gliding through the corridors. Like ghosts emerging from the walls and tunnels. I felt like I was part of a large commercial enterprise. The pharmacists and scientists made the drug and then it was dispersed to the doctors, a small business, then to me the consumer. I would pay for the services through my insurance company, keeping the pharmacies and specialised doctors in employment. My main duty was to ingest the product.

They must have a patent on mental illness.

I felt like I wanted to take all my clothes off, sit waiting at the nurses' station and see the shock on their faces.

Would they notice that? It would be inappropriate behaviour and would certainly give them something to do or think about. Perhaps not, because they would be used to that and it would only give them grounds to make me ingest more of their product.

I saw Celia bouncing towards me, her hips swinging. They looked out of proportion to the rest of her body.

She was talking to another nurse. 'I know they're using the system, because they don't try and get better' do they?' said Celia.

'They just complain all the time,' the other nurse said. 'I wish they'd do something to help themselves. It's not a hostel, it's a hospital.' The other nurse was also short and had a nose that was similar to a parrot.

Doesn't she know I can hear them? Surely they could be a bit more compassionate. They're nurses. Who would want to stay here for the fun of it?

'Gardenia, there you are.' Celia's dark eyes, gleaming teeth and hooked nose stared at me. I felt sorry for her. She needed a good night's sleep or plastic surgery.

You're a toad. The voice had returned.

I knew my diagnosis. I had an inferiority complex with identity issues and a guilt complex as an extra bonus. I felt angry with myself for thinking I had a problem.

I can't help it if she's ugly. It's not my fault, is it?

'I'll be back in a minute,' Celia said.

Well, I'm not going anywhere. Just as well, otherwise we'd never catch up?

I waited. Celia took five minutes, which felt like two hours. When she came back, she unlocked the door to the nurses' station and I watched her fossick about in a cupboard.

'Baxter, now let me see if I can find you. Under B, isn't it?'

I hoped she wouldn't find me in the cupboard, if she did, my recovery would be jeopardised. Celia took out the small tray carrying the varied medications that I was to ingest. 'You have the risperdal this morning too and the alprazolam, five milligrams.'

She pressed out the small pills into a plastic cup. 'You're starting the antidepressant this morning too. The effexor, I've heard very good reports about this one.'

I wasn't going to disagree.

She placed the cup under the glass window. 'The water fountain is just there and, Gardenia, could you keep the plastic cup, it helps with the recycling.'

Does she mean I have to carry a plastic cup around with me?

'Why don't you put our names on the cups and stand them in a line near the window?' I said.

'That's an interesting idea. You should bring that up in the meetings.'

'You have meetings here, like political stuff,' I said. *Can I take this regime over?*

I swallowed the tablets and water in one gulp.

'I'll do your blood pressure now,' said Celia.

'Do you take it everyday?' I said.

She nodded.

I sat in the same chair as she wheeled the blood pressure machine towards me. She placed the stretchy material around my upper arm. The machine made buzzing and beeping noises.

'Stand up now,' Celia said.

I looked at the numbers on the machine. Celia didn't say anything, so it was probable that my blood pressure was normal. Although it could have been sky rocketing and she didn't want to frighten me.

'Why do you have to take the blood pressure twice?' I asked.

'Because when you stand up quickly, your blood pressure can drop.'

'Does that mean I can't play sport? Is that because of the side effects of the medication?' It was the first time I had mentioned the words 'side effect' to a member of the medical Gestapo. I knew they didn't believe in such terminology but this was a private hospital. *Maybe they have different standards.*

'Some of your medication can do that, especially when you first start an antidepressant, but it's rare.'

'I suppose you have to be methodical, if you don't want people to die.'

'That's right.'

'But what's the point of having medication that can make you ill?'

'All medication has side effects.'

Her reinforcement of my theory made me nearly pass out. I thought better of it, as she'd blame my blood pressure and I'd have to take another tablet.

'You're telling me. I think it slows down my thinking, that's why I'm depressed.'

'Isn't it better to take something to relieve your thoughts?'

'Yes, but that doesn't happen, does it? I only have depression, and that's because of my thoughts.' I felt like saying it was the mental health system that made me depressed.

'What other things have been happening to you? Have you been feeling paranoid?'

I chose not to answer that question. 'The medications have made me constipated,' I said.

'We can give you something for that.'

'I'm not having an enema. I don't think I've been for a week. I'm not having them stick detergent up there again.'

'No, we won't do that. We have nu lax,' Celia said as if it would cure all known bowel problems.

'Isn't there something else I can take – it doesn't work.'

I don't know why I was asking for her opinion. My previous theoretical discussions with chemists in regards to bowel movements had proved futile. Did they have any other mechanical means of eliminating toxins?

I felt like I could write a thesis on the use of suppositories and other anal extraction materials.

'We have that nice orange drink, Metamucil,' Celia said.

Does it fizz? We could make a fortune selling it to kids pretending it was a new pop drink.

'That doesn't work either. A laxette might help.' The old proven method was always the better option.

'No, I don't think there appropriate. They're addictive,' said Celia.

'Addictive? You mean I'll have withdrawal symptoms? I'll want to take them all the time?'

'No, I mean your bowels will become lazy, or slow.'

'They're already slow. I don't think it'll make much difference.'

'Your muscles will eventually lose their power to push, so to speak.'

I felt like I had just been diagnosed with bowel cancer. I wondered if I should tell the nurse about my urinating problems. Although I didn't want to hear that I might have cancer of the bladder.

'How are you feeling generally?' Celia changed the subject.

'What, with a lazy bowel?'

'No, your general health.'

'Bloody lousy.'

'Can you define lousy?'

'I don't have a dictionary.'

'No, I mean can you say a bit more about how you're feeling, like what you're thinking?'

'Well, I'm trying to make judgements in my head. Sorting the wheat from the chaff is problematic. There are many rooms in my mansion.' *Does that sound psychotic?*

'Many rooms?' said Celia.

'Yes, and I go to prepare one for you. I don't know what you expect me to say. I can't figure it out. It's the medication. I'm on too much. I can't think properly and I hear my own thoughts.'

'You're hearing your thoughts?'

'Yes, but they're not voices, like hallucinations. I know they're my thoughts.'

'I see. Do they bother you? Do you feel anxious?'

'I don't know what I feel. I don't think the antidepressants are working.'

'You've just started them, Gardenia. You have to be patient. The doctor will help you.'

She could probably do a better job than you, I thought.

'I'm not having electric therapy again. I've just got my memory back, I think. Is it correct that you lose your short-term memory for six months after ECT?'

'Yes, that's right,' said Celia.

I nearly passed out again. She was agreeing with me. I knew now that I wasn't sick.

There isn't anything wrong with me. It's their tablets.

'When am I seeing my doctor?' I said.

'Just a moment, I'll check.' Celia went to the nurses' station. 'Your doctor's going to see you tomorrow and the general practitioner's going to see you today.'

'Witch doctor?' I said. I thought the term was appropriate.

'I'll let you know when Dr Jarvie arrives. The medical doctor will be here soon.'

Not more tests.

'When are visiting times?' I asked. I wondered if my mother was going to visit me today.

'Any time, and your visitor can stop for a meal too, but they have to pay a small fee,' she said.

'Really. I'll have to ring up Mum and invite her for tea.'

'That's a good idea. The phones are just in there.' Celia pointed down the hallway.

I went to room number twenty-three and took some coins from my purse. I went to the red phone and rang my home number.

'Hello, Mum, it's me.'

'Gardenia, how are you?'

I knew she was sad but putting on a brave front. 'Are you all right?' I said.

'Yes, I'm okay. Are you all right?'

This is getting repetitive.

'Are they treating you okay?'

'Better than I expected,' I said. 'Put it this way, I don't feel like I'm a list of symptoms. I mean, they haven't placed me in a pigeonhole.' *Or a cell for that matter.*

'That's good to hear,' she said.

'I think they're weird, the doctors and nurses. I mean, to be continually looking for mental delusions. I wouldn't find that very inspiring, would you? It would get me down after a while. If you could cure people, it wouldn't be so bad, would it?'

'No, I suppose not,' my mother said.

'It's not a case of treating a headache, is it? At least that goes away, hopefully. If I wasn't making my patients better, I'd give up. Or at least try something different. Having patients locked up or sedated isn't very useful, is it? I wonder if they enjoy what they do. It's about time someone did something about treating us like human beings. I'm not a stupid moron, am I?'

'No, Gardenia, I don't think you are. No one's saying that, are they?'

'No, but I'm sure they're thinking it. Perhaps I should form a cult like the Masons. The moronic group, or we-haven't-got-a-bloody-clue club or something? Are you coming in today to visit? The nurse said you can have a meal here.'

'I might not come in today, Gardenia. My legs are aching and I'm not walking properly.'

'Probably the heat, Mum. You'll feel better soon. Just rest, okay? It's quite nice here. I'm seeing the doctor tomorrow. It's better than Felixstowe, isn't it? At least I see a doctor. They have plenty of chairs here too. I don't have to fight with other patients just to sit down. That's something, isn't it? Plus I can go to my bedroom any time I like.'

'Yes, that is very good. I'll see how I feel tomorrow.'

'Okay, Mum, but if you're not up to it, please stay at home and rest. I'll ring you tomorrow. I love you, Mum.'

I went outside to the garden. I sat on a bench and stared at the fountain.

It comprised a stone statue of a young girl, naked, holding a jug to her breast. I watched the unrelenting water erupting from the urn like a mini waterfall. I tried to focus on its power, hoping its energy would flow through the tributaries in my veins, purifying and cleansing, eliminating toxins.

I studied the bees hovering over the lavender bush. The blue purplish flowers contrasted against the deep green leaves. I looked at the jasmine vine and its delicate white flowers creeping around the pillars of the bull nose veranda. I could see the tendrils stretching out to find an anchor, so it could continue to grow. *At least the plant has its freedom to live. What chance have I got?*

I wanted to leave, to break free from this prison. I remembered running away from Felixstowe, catching the tram, not having any money to buy the ticket and the bus conductor saying 'God help us all.' I remembered the high security ward.

I could say I'm okay, thanks, and discharge myself. I could see another doctor, tell him I'm not mad, but it would be hard to deny a professional doctor's opinion.

I remembered parts of the conversation I had earlier with the voices in my mind. They told me I was a star and they adored me. Then they made fun of me. I wanted to believe that the voices were my own thoughts, delusions created to combat previous trauma. If I didn't understand myself, try to make sense of my mind in a realistic or rational manner, then I'd be doomed to live out the rest of my life in a mental institution. I was aware of the fantastical nature of my hallucinations and my inability to control my unconscious mind.

Is it my response to alleviate mental anguish? Is it my way of coping with harsh treatment? My imagination exploring alternatives to be better understood? So I can be treated with love and care. Am I just pretending, talking to imaginary characters? Perhaps it's a symptom of my pent-up frustration with others not understanding me?

Then there was the depressing side to having voices that were not friendly. To hear the cruel words and abuse, the morbid distressing ideas and confusing motives, the humiliation.

I can't tell the doctors that they're wrong. I'm dependent on a system. I found it hard to accept this fact. I didn't like the continuing analysis, the ever-continuing medication, the sleeplessness, the anxiety and the anger. I felt helpless and longed for sanity, a way of living that was not such hard work. I felt persecuted, as if I was living in a depressing saga of a mad soap opera with nowhere to go. I had fallen off a star and was lost in space. It didn't matter if the cushion covers of the sofa were made of threads of gold – I was still a woman locked in a cage.

I saw an older woman sitting on a wicker chair, under the veranda. I thought about making conversation. I could acknowledge her with a greeting, say it was a lovely day. But then what was lovely about it?

A nurse ventured out into the sunlight. She carried a clipboard and wrote down some notes, checking the patients and doing her rounds.

Perhaps I could say I'm not here.

'Don't drink too much of that coffee, Libby. You won't sleep tonight,' the efficient nurse said to the older woman.

'I don't think it's just the coffee that's keeping me awake,' she replied.

I realised that I wasn't the only one with a sleep disorder. Libby's hair looked like it had wrestled with a tornado, been ripped off and then plonked back on her head.

The woman noticed me staring at her. 'I haven't seen you before. Who's your doctor?' she said.

'Dr Jarvie,' I replied.

'Oh yes,' the woman drawled, breathing in her cigarette, followed by a hacking cough. 'What medication are you taking and is it working?'

I wondered if she wanted medical advice; if so, she was speaking to the wrong person.

'I don't know if it's working but I'm taking haloperidol, tegretol and lithium. No, I'm wrong. I'm taking perphenazine, orphenadrine, lorazepam and temazepam. No, I'm not telling the truth, they've just been changed and I'm taking risperdal, effexor, alprazolam and I don't think I'm taking a mood stabiliser. Oh yes I am, but I can't remember.'

'You've done well so far,' Libby said. 'I give you credit for having a good memory. But whatever you're taking, it sounds like a cocktail. You don't want to take that haloperidol for too long. How long have you been taking it?'

'Six years.' I couldn't forget my age, when I was first admitted to Felixstowe at twenty-one.

'It's a bad drug. I've seen the damage it's caused. The side effects give you a shaking disease like Parkinson's.'

'Is that why I've been having tremors?' I said.

'Yes. It also makes people continually pace. It can make you rigid as well, like your face becomes immobile like a wax dummy.'

I remembered the times when I couldn't stop my legs from moving, constantly restless and agitated. When my head lolled to one side and I couldn't move it.

'How do they know these things work, or are we the test cases?' I said.

'Well, they certainly can't find schizophrenia in chimpanzees, can they?'

'I thought it was all part of my illness, like it was my fault,' I said.

'Oh no, dear, those are the side effects.' The woman coughed again. She banged her chest. 'I must give these things up, but not while I'm in hospital. The nicotine helps my brain. Anyway, that's my excuse. Don't worry, you're young – you'll get better,' she added.

I saw a man sitting in the far corner of the garden, watching me. He was fair-haired and slim and wore round black-rimmed glasses. I could feel his eyes penetrating my mind and his thoughts connecting with mine. He was taking me hostage.

I know you can't do this. His voice was loud in my mind. *I can overcome all evil but you will always remain insane.*

I'm not insane, you are, I replied. *I can overcome this because I am logical. I will never give in.*

But I have strength far superior to yours. I have the power to take control. His voice was hard. I had to remain sane.

No, you don't, I replied. *I can overcome any insanity that you would like to throw at me. Got it?*

I felt like I had won. My mind was battling against unreal forces. My only hope was to fight and I could not rest until the battle was over. I watched the man get up and walk into another part of the hospital.

'Have you ever been to Felixstowe?' I asked Libby.

'Only once, thankfully. Why? Have you been there?'

'Yes, I was in there for six months.'

Libby didn't say anything. She stubbed out her cigarette and lit another one.

'I was in a sexual molesters' ward for a time,' I said.

Libby looked at me and I'm sure she was impressed.

I remembered the Arabic man and an old man who looked like Burl Ives, the country and western singer. Why did I allow the old man to touch me? I must have been sedated. I visualised the nurse in the secure ward. He liked to fondle my breasts too. Did he really think he was helping me?

'My mother rang the media, because I was getting molested. I had a nurse by my side twenty-four hours a day after that,' I said.

'I'm not surprised,' Libby said.

'They let me go home after that,' I said.

I tried to remember what we'd been talking about before I mentioned being molested. *It was about side effects, wasn't it?*

'Can antipsychotics give you epilepsy?' I asked.

'I knew a person who kept on having epileptic fits and when they changed his tablets, he didn't have another,' Libby said and she looked into her cigarette packet. 'Guess I'll have to get more of these.'

Suddenly I heard a loud bell ringing.

'The place isn't on fire, that's the meal time bell. Lunch is served,' said Libby.

I joined the long queue of patients waiting for their meals in the dining room. *God, I'm even forced to eat. Maybe they're getting us fat for their experiments.*

I looked around and was sure some of the patients looked like guinea pigs. Then guinea pigs eat lettuce, don't they?

I took a plate of salad back to my usual spot near the exit door.

Celia found me again in the dining room. 'I think it would be good to have a session or a short discussion, just to find out how you're coping. Do you think that's a good idea?'

Do I have a choice?

I nodded.

'Let's find a vacant room, shall we?'

I had finished my small salad and followed Celia down the hallway. She opened a door. 'This is the relaxation room,' she said.

I saw a large black chair standing in the middle of the room.

'That massage chair is great if you can't sleep. It has a rhythm. See, here's the remote control. You can change it to the strength you need. It's especially good for aching muscles too.'

An electric chair. Great, I thought.

We then went into the next room along the hall. It was another consulting room. We sat opposite each other on floral cushioned armchairs.

'Have you settled in?' She looked at her notes. She didn't wait for a reply. 'How have you been feeling?'

'I think I'm depressed.'

'It's a terrible feeling. Mind you, I've never experienced real deep depression.'

'Yes, but I know why I'm depressed,' I said.

'Oh yes?' Celia looked intrigued.

'Because I can't think properly or put my mind on anything positive.'

'Well, that's a start to be aware of that. It's a symptom of depression, slowed-down thinking. Perhaps you'd like to work in our craft room. There are lots of things to do.'

I did not want to accept myself as a mad person with disabilities, the stigma of being 'not altogether there'. I wanted to deny that sort of judgement. I certainly didn't want to paint ceramic objects, like we had at Felixstowe.

'It would take your mind off your problems. Perhaps you could paint what you're feeling?'

I didn't have the interest or capacity to want to paint or draw. I had thought about painting. Expressing my feelings and how they could be translated into art work. I was sure it would be very abstract, an image symbolic of making connections, like cracks in a stone pavement. Or perhaps I could paint a black canvas, with a very small dot of white in the middle? I could call it *Hope*. My art work would probably take on proportions of something very depressing, like demonic faces. That subject would not help my anxiety, or depression for that matter.

Suddenly I felt sorry for the nurse, the patients, the doctors, everyone in the mental health system; in fact, everyone on the planet. They were only trying to help and they weren't doing that very well.

'It would help you to relax. Distraction is a good way of overcoming irrational thinking.'

'But I can't remember what I did yesterday at two p.m.'

'Oh, everyone can't remember everything. If we did, we wouldn't be normal. We'd all end up in a place like this.'

I wonder if she's aware of what she's saying.

A voice in my mind spoke. Who needs enemies when you have friends like that? She's a narrow-minded, insecure bitch who enjoys humiliating others. She just wants to upset you. There's no reason why you should stay. Just go and pack your bags and leave. I would.

But I could get worse. I can't go off the medication cold turkey. These chemicals are dangerous, they alter your thoughts. I could get very sick.

What's the alternative? Stay here for the rest of your days?

I'll leave but then they'll send me back to hospital. Next time I'll be locked up. I don't want to go back there again, to Felixstowe.

Don't worry. I'll be with you, the voice trailed off.

Another voice entered my mind. The speech had a different tonal quality. Hello, I'm a doctor. I don't think you should take that young man's opinion seriously. If you disregard your current doctor, you may have to find another. The notes will be passed on and they'll make their own judgement, probably increasing the antipsychotic. They'll make a realistic assumption based on prior treatment. You can't live under that sort of pressure, continually challenging the medical system.

I was aware of the nurse staring at me. 'I was just thinking about the tablets. That perhaps I'm on too much.'

'Your doctor has you on this medication for a reason. I can't judge whether it's right to decrease the tablets. Perhaps you should talk to your doctor.' Celia had a worried brow.

I knew she thought I was preoccupied with hearing voices. She was right, but I couldn't let her know that.

What's the point of talking to them? a voice in my mind said. *They just say you're paranoid, delusional, for even thinking to oppose their ideas.*

'Perhaps you need some medication now,' said Celia. 'Everyone has a certain predisposition towards suffering a psychosis. It depends on the amount of stress a person goes through. Some are more susceptible than others.'

She realises that I can't hold a conversation.

We went back to the nurses' station.

Celia gave me a small blue pill. 'That's your alprazolam. It'll help with the anxiety. The GP's here. Just sit outside the end consulting room and he'll be with you in a minute.'

I naturally thought that a doctor was supposed to help a person's health and I thought if I resisted, it would be a 'non-normal' thing to do. I waited for the GP.

A young man in his thirties opened the door. He had black hair, wore a suit and didn't smile. He looked serious. 'Gardenia Baxter?' he said.

'Yes.'

'Please come in.'

The room had a desk and a chair next to the desk.

He pointed to the chair. 'Please take a seat.'

I watched him as he looked through my file. He studied it for a short time.

'Have you had any major illnesses, operations?'

'Yes, a termination a few years ago.'

'Any history of blood pressure, diabetes?'

'I remember my father having high blood pressure and my mother has type 2 diabetes, mature onset.'

'Both your mother and father are still alive?'

'My father died when I was young, a heart attack. My mother is still alive.'

I watched him write down these answers. I looked around the room. There was an examination bed covered with a white sheet, a board with letters in various sizes was on the wall, a blood pressure machine stood near the bed. Everything was clean and clinical, typical of a general practitioner's consulting room.

'Can you sit up on the bed there.'

I did and he placed the stethoscope on my chest and back, asking me to breathe deeply.

'Can you lie down now.'

He used a small rubber stick and tapped the appropriate places, my ankles, knees, elbows, to see if my reflexes were working.

'Can you just pull down your jeans, so I can feel your stomach.'

I knew the procedure and understood he was carrying out a general examination.

He pressed around my stomach and I thought I saw him frown, just for a moment.

'Okay, that will be all. You can get down now.'

'I can leave then?'

'Yes, that's fine.'

I smiled at him and said thank you.

He didn't respond and went back to his desk to continue writing his notes.

I went outside to the garden again. I didn't want to stay in my room, battling with my thoughts. The garden was the only place where I had some freedom from my anxiety. I could try to relax, if that was at all possible. It was a safe place, but I resented it. Happiness was a thing I could only fleetingly remember. Had the tempest blown over? I was unsure and that made me agitated. I was living in a war zone, ready to jump, to escape. I was exhausted.

I saw Libby sitting outside. I went over and sat next to her, under the shelter of the veranda, away from the hot sun.

'What dot are you on?' said Libby.

I'm not on a dot, am I? I looked down at the ground, at my feet. *I can't see any dots. Is she seeing dots?*

'Don't you know about the dots?' Libby said.

I shook my head.

'A red dot means you can't leave the premises. A green dot means you can leave on your own, but you always have to tell the nurses where you're going and when you'll be back. You better talk to the nurse if you don't know what dot you're on.'

'Is there an orange dot?'

'Yes, that means you can leave but only with a responsible adult,' said Libby.

I didn't like the idea of being detained.

'The Red Cross come every Wednesday and you can have a manicure or facial. There's also the shopping complex up the street. You can go there if you're on a green dot.'

'This is certainly different to Felixstowe,' I said. I felt like I had a bad case of the measles.

'I wouldn't put my dog in there,' Libby said. 'Do you like writing? I find it useful, to recognise my emotions and watch for triggers. Sometimes I think I should be working. I really would like paid employment, but I just keep on getting sick. Anyway who would want to employ a mentally ill person with a drug problem? If you weren't in here for depression, you soon would be.'

I was depressed by Libby's conversation, but I wasn't going to tell her that.

I looked at Libby's head. *Perhaps if you combed your hair you might feel better? God, what am I saying? I am so superficial.*

We sat in silence. I didn't talk about my problems. I didn't want to increase her depression, or mine for that matter. I had made a decision. My diagnosis was depression. It sounded reasonable. I wanted to ask Libby what her diagnosis was, but thought it was too personal. I disliked the idea of generalising and judging another person's discomfort, with meaningless assumptions. It was a human condition to categorise and make meaning with labels in an effort to understand. Classifying people, judging them, wasn't really helpful. It had its limitations. *Perhaps I could ask her if she's a pony or a racehorse.*

I saw another patient enter the garden. He was wearing a light blue dressing gown with printed images of black skulls. The belt of his robe was dragging beside him and his slippers were far too large for him. I watched him shuffle with his arms straight at his sides. He reminded me of a zombie. He walked around the fountain, turning in a circular fashion and then went back into the building.

'Perhaps he's practising an eastern meditation,' I said.

'I don't think so,' replied Libby.

I remembered the time in Felixstowe, in the secure ward, the large white linoleum floor and the nurses watching me as I moved my body in jerking spasms. I wanted to ask Libby if the choreographic movements I was making were caused by medication. *Would she know?*

I decided to go to the television room and watch the news. I saw murder, rape, people lying and committing fraud. People saying criminals should be locked up forever and victims were not getting justice. I was sickened with horror because I knew I was the perpetrator. After all, I had been locked up. I was the one who was weird and should be ostracised. I was not pleased about feeling this way and it made me blame the victim's family. *God, they're weak, why can't they cope with a murdered friend?* I realised it was an absurd and horrifying thought. *Perhaps I'm the cruel person, the one who is a criminal.*

I remembered the night when I walked home in the dark from a friend's place. I thought someone was following me and I ran into a nearby house. I was scared, thinking I was going to be murdered. I was eventually taken home in a police paddy wagon. I was still unsure if it was due to my paranoia or if I was being followed.

Maybe it has something to do with my past, the movies I watched as a teenager. The real-life horror stories of women getting raped and murdered by some sexual deviant. I was scared of my own mental fragility, wondering if I had the capability of being a sociopathic killer.

I've just watched the five o'clock news, that's all. It's enough to make anyone traumatised.

I took my medication early, as I wanted to go to bed, to sleep, perchance to dream. It was the best part of my day. Even if I did have horrific nightmares, I didn't remember them. The electric therapy had helped in that regard. Eighteen days of sleep deprivation had made me realise the importance of rapid eye movement. I knew if my unconscious mind did not dream, make symbols and odd connections, then my brain would need an alternative, to reboot the system, so to speak. My conscious mind would dream and I would be aware of it. I did not want to step into that world again.

During the night, I had disturbing dreams. I was lost, running down hallways or tunnels. I saw a small rabbit caught in a trap, crying with pain, trying to escape. I could hear a wailing noise. The animal was fighting and I saw the steel blades cut deeper into the skin. Then I watched the small body decompose rapidly into the earth. Then I found myself in a room, with a shiny white linoleum floor. I could feel the cold substance under my bare feet. I saw myself signing papers as I watched a girl move in acrobatic ways, jerking and pushing her body, in strange directions. The girl was gesturing with her arms, creating a story with her body, turning, running on the spot.

The images shifted and I could see faces contorted in terror looking through small windows. I could see that they were screaming, but I could not hear them. More images came into my mind. I saw my spindly body, naked and hunched over, sitting on a plastic chair. A long line of men were watching me. I could see people behind a large pane of glass, looking at me. There was another image of a man dressed in pyjamas. He didn't have any fingers. He comforted me, telling me not to be afraid, because he could not strangle me. Another man was making a buzzing noise. It began as a quiet low hum and gradually increased in volume. The dream changed and I saw the rabbit again, scratching a hole under a barbed-wire fence. I tried to summon all my telepathic power to aid in its escape.

When I awoke, I remembered this nightmare. I knew it had not been a dream. It had happened.

3

Next morning after breakfast and medication, I asked the staff for some paper. I then went back to my room to try and write. Libby's idea of expression through creative writing sounded promising. If I could explain myself in words, perhaps it would make me feel better.

My scribbling contained ideas and jumbled descriptive passages outlining my state of mind. I tried to concentrate on the words in front of me. I wanted this expression to be a form of therapy but instead it made me more distressed. *How can I explain my thoughts when I can't even think?*

I felt like I was a contradiction in terms, wanting to ignore or change my situation and then examining it, to the point of obsession. I felt like I was in an hourglass and was perpetually being turned upside down. The grains were always the same, but the thoughts were continually mixed. Like a timeless prison.

I had heard of 'stream of consciousness' writing. Perhaps using it, I could figure out the underlying cause of my illness. I started writing quickly without constraint.

I am hibernating, so I can sleep to make myself fresh. I am living in a dream world. The past is still with me but I have this purpose on earth to be a saint. Or am I an angel wrapped in some disused clothes? It's only an outer appearance so I can help others? Am I connected to anything else? Which way do I go? Should I jump from right to left? Can I go backwards and forwards? Can change happen with movement and line? Yes, it's transformation.

Trying to understand myself was a courageous act. I felt that my logical or intelligent mind had vaporised a long time ago.

I could make myself feel better by fantasising, thinking my life had purpose. If I had a publishing contract, I could use my experiences and journal writings for something constructive, perhaps a book to help others? I imagined myself sitting in a French bistro in the countryside, writing my new bestseller, whilst drinking a glass of vintage red. I was a successful writer, happy and fulfilled.

Who in their right mind would publish my weirdo thoughts.

I left my incoherent ideas and went outside to the garden again, hoping a change in scenery would transform me. I saw a young man dressed in a white T-shirt and black pants. His face looked familiar and I recognised him from yesterday. He was the patient who had been walking like a zombie. He was a different person. *How could he have changed in so little time? What medication had he been given?*

I looked at him and he looked at me. His bright blue eyes were piercing and alarming.

He strode up to me and nonchalantly smiled. 'Hello. I haven't seen you before. I would have remembered that.'

Oh God, I'm in some deviant type of Mills and Boon book. I wondered if was his way of coping, to be so nice. After all, we were in a very different, irregular and unusual environment. Or was his outgoing personality a part of his condition? *Is he manic?*

Suddenly a young girl flew out the door. She knocked the pot plant that was sitting on the banister to the ground. 'Oh, bloody hell,' she said.

'Don't worry, they'll clean it up afterwards,' the man in the white T-shirt said.

The girl looked at him in disgust as if his opinion wasn't warranted. She heaved a big sigh and lit a cigarette. She looked at me with suspicion. 'I don't want to be here! Do you understand? Does anyone hear me?' the girl cried. 'Why am I here?'

I was conscious of my own apathy and felt guilty. *Wisdom is supposed to come with age.*

'It'll be okay,' I said, trying to assuage the girl's fear.

'It'll be okay? Locked up in a loony bin, trying to find out if you're sane? Wanting a future, wanting anything? Sure!'

The young man went to the girl and sat beside her. 'Do you mind if I sit next to you?' he asked.

At least he has manners.

'No, and if you don't mind, bugger off,' the girl said.

Well, she certainly doesn't have manners. God, where was she brought up?

'Why am I here? Am I insane? I'm not taking their bloody pills!' The girl's eyes were like huge staring dark circles.

The man with the blue eyes was going to be persistent. 'It is a bit bewildering, isn't it? Don't worry, we're all insane here,' he said, as if that explained everything.

The girl looked at him in shock. Then she suddenly laughed. It was a high-toned shrill. 'You know, this is really funny,' she cried.

'I know,' said the man.

'I mean, we're all nuts. They tell us we're nuts, and then we're given pills and told to use self-help or whatever. Then we go home. I reckon they're nuts.' She was starting to enjoy herself.

'Oh, no, I don't think they're nuts. They're making too much money,' he said. 'I'm leaving tomorrow, although I could stay another couple of days, if you wanted me around,' he added.

'Why would I want you around?' the girl said and they looked at each other and burst into laughter.

'We could have a good time,' he said. I could tell he was trying not to burst into laughter again. 'We've got coffee here for free, and we can talk.'

'Good God, you are insane.'

Again they reeled into laughter. I could understand the humour, but I didn't think it was that funny. I was envious of them. Two complete strangers, comfortable together, sharing a joke. I didn't want to join in the conversation so I looked intently at the fountain, pretending it was of great interest to me.

'Are you okay?' the blue-eyed man said.

I realised he was talking to me.

'Yes, I'm just meditating.'

'What sort of meditation?' he asked.

'It's the one where you look at something for a very long time,' said the girl.

'Really?' he said.

'It's like daydreaming,' I explained.

'Oh, really? And what sort of dreams do you see?' he said.

A male nurse came out and walked up to us. He forced his large bottom into one of the wicker chairs. He grinned. 'Having fun?' he said.

The young man and girl burst into laughter again. I wondered if I should go and get a piece of paper and pencil and draw the fountain.

'So what do you know?' the nurse said.

'Not much,' the man said. 'I wanted to talk to you.' The blue-eyed man looked like he was getting ready for a deep and meaningful conversation. He placed his large cup of coffee on top of the brick wall that surrounded the veranda and lit a cigarette.

'Yeah, sure. Do you want to go inside where it's more private?' said the nurse.

'No, it's okay. I've got nothing to hide.' He looked at the young girl and smiled.

'Yes, but if it's personal…' the nurse continued.

'Well, I think we're all in the same boat, don't you think?' He then gave the girl a wink.

I felt like telling the girl to beware of men like him, but I realised the young woman could look after herself.

'Okay, what's on your mind, Guy? How can I help?'

What a question? You can bloody get us out of here, I thought.

'Aren't you supposed to know what's wrong with me?' said Guy.

The nurse looked at Guy quizzically. 'Have you been feeling upset about your home life? I remember you telling me you wanted to move out,' he said.

Well, this isn't a conversation about psychosis. It's an everyday chat. How weird.

The young woman had decided to walk around the garden. She picked a few daisies and I wondered if she was going to say, 'He loves me, he loves me not'?

'I don't know why I'm here,' Guy said. 'I've been trying to answer that question all my life. Well, not all the time, but it has been an interest of mine. Existential matters, the afterlife, or parallel worlds. It's very interesting, isn't it?' he continued. 'Do you know why you're here? Anyway, I'm not crazy, if that's what you think.'

No one here gives a direct answer, or one that makes sense.

'Although I have been thinking about the community housing project,' said Guy.

I looked at the nurse. He reminded me of a leech. His face was red and puffy and he had a thick neck, as wide as his head. I could see him stuck to a wall and the other nurses trying to scrape him off. I shook my head to try and dispel the image.

'Can you find out about it?' said Guy.

'Yeah, sure. When I've got some information, I'll find you and we can talk about it. Other than that, are you okay?'

He got out of that one easily.

'I hate some people,' said Guy.

The girl in the garden giggled.

'Oh, and why is that?'

I thought the poor man was being investigated by an alien leech.

'People are a bunch of selfish users. I try to help and they take the shirt off my back.'

'Who are these people?' said the nurse.

'My friends, those I hang around with.'

The girl looked up, spread out her arms and jumped up and down on the spot.

'They can't be good friends.'

'No, they're not. I don't have proper friends. I don't have any friends. They're like vultures. As soon as they see some vulnerability, they pounce. It's as if I'm a bit of roadkill.'

'Roadkill?'

Obviously nurse leech has no idea

'Yes, bloody roadkill.' Guy emphasised this by putting his hand to his throat and mimicking a knife slashed his neck.

'Oh, I see,' said the nurse.

'I'm so bloody generous, you know,' Guy continued. 'I'm kind, to the point of having nothing left. I thought I had a friend in Mike, and we could have a good time together, going out and having a few drinks. Well, he let me down too.'

'How did he let you down?'

'He just wanted to sell me his clothes, second-hand stuff that was worn!'

I could sense Guy was getting angry.

'I'm always giving away my cigarettes, because that's what friends do, don't they? Then they expect me to do things for them. Go to the shop, get them this or that from the chemist, the list goes on.'

He is definitely getting overwhelmed.

'Okay,' the nurse said. 'Perhaps it's good to see these things in perspective. Discovering what you want and what you don't want is a positive thing. So look for new and better friends. Find people who are supportive and can give something back.'

'Okay, but how do I do that?'

'There are courses and groups, where you can just sit and chat over coffee. Try and find something you like doing. Having things in common helps a friendship blossom.'

Did he really say 'blossom'? I laughed and I wondered if they could hear my thoughts.

'Oh no, not more craft groups. I don't want to play chess, or do cooking, or bingo, or art class.'

Art class might not be so bad. I wondered if it would help me.

I looked at Guy. He was like a tight coil ready to jump and I thought he might possibly leap off his chair.

'So you don't mean going down the pub and getting drunk, then going home with a mate, to wake up next morning and find everything of importance you own gone?'

I was impressed with his long-winded sentence.

'Yes, that's just what I mean. Find other ways of forming friendships. Do you think you're worthy of a good friendship?'

I saw the girl now lying flat on the concrete lifting her legs up and down. I wondered why I didn't have any friends.

'Yes, of course I'm capable of being a friend. I just haven't been lucky.'

61

'Those friendships are boring,' the girl said. 'Anyway you have to be a friend to have a friend.'

I was surprised with the young woman's nonchalance. Did she hate this place or did she really care if she was in a mental home? I watched her getting up and down, seemingly unable to make up her mind whether to remain lying down, jumping on the spot or was she going to climb up the sandstone wall? I hoped she wasn't going to jump in the fountain. *She could knock her head and then the ambulance will arrive. They'll ask me questions. They might think I did it in an act of rage.*

'It's not a matter of luck, it's your choice, but understanding how you want to be treated is a great first move,' the nurse continued.

'And now, my landlord is thinking of kicking me out, only because he found some cigarette burns on the carpet. Now he says I have to smoke outside,' said Guy.

That's pretty harsh treatment. Doesn't he pay rent?

'But he's not going to kick you out then?' the nurse said.

'No, but he will, if I don't smoke outside.'

Does this nurse understand? You don't need to be a Rhodes scholar to figure it out.

'I'll have to sit on a stool in my garage which has nothing in it and look at the tin galvanised sheeting all day,' Guy said. 'That won't be a lot of fun.'

'Don't you have an outdoor area?'

Yeah, with a swimming pool, sauna and deckchairs.

'Yes, but what happens if it's raining?' Guy was starting to look tired.

Stand under an umbrella? It's not that difficult to work out, is it? People pay good money to come in here and talk about these things. I wondered if I was the only one on the planet who had some sense.

'Maybe the community housing project isn't such a bad idea,' the nurse said.

'I know. That's what I told you in the first place,' Guy said.

He gets paid for this, but then only someone getting paid would listen to this ranting.

I looked at the nurse with new respect. I tried to ignore their conversation, which was not an easy thing to do. I turned to the girl, who had now calmed down and was sitting next to me. She was lighting a cigarette.

'Aren't they wonderful, those big ghost gums?' I pointed upwards to the farthest corner of the hospital.

'Yes, and isn't it a wonderful day?' said the girl.

I wanted to say that she was a rude spoilt child and should be drowned in the nearest fountain, but then I felt sorry for her, and then guilty because I had thought of murder, and then felt paranoid that I would be sent to prison because of it.

'They remind you of those Hans Heysen paintings, don't they?' I said. I was not going to be thwarted by the girl's ignorance.

'Hans who?' the girl said and showed her distaste by spitting into the shrubbery.

'The gums, they look old and timeless.'

'They're just gum trees. God, get it together,' the girl said.

I decided to focus my attention on Guy's conversation with nurse leech. I also realised that it wasn't the four walls that made this hospital a prison. It was the uncomfortable surroundings, being confined with difficult personalities.

'Maybe someone could help me for a change? Or should I take care of myself more?' Guy said.

'That's an interesting point,' said the nurse.

'I could earn it. I could pay my way. I could clean, do something. That's how I could raise my self-esteem. Maybe someone would value me. Recognise me?'

I felt like I was in a television talk show.

'I know it's hard to find friends, but true friends are few and far between,' said nurse leech.

'I end up binge drinking at hotels, because I panic when it comes to socialising and those same patterns keep on bringing me back to hospital.'

Guy is certainly humiliating himself. He should have gone in and spoken privately.

'When I get drunk, I get angry. Once I caused property damage and had to spend a night in gaol.'

'Oh, we all do that. Get over it,' said the girl.

'There are always alternatives,' said the nurse. 'I'll see you tomorrow and perhaps we can work out a plan. Maybe you could think of some relaxing things you would like to do?'

'Enjoyable things?' said Guy.

I was getting sick and tired of listening to Guy's relentless moaning. I thought about going somewhere else, hiding in my room, but then it made me angry, that I should be the one to leave. *Why can't I stay here and have some peace and quiet?* My attempts to rationalise my emotions failed.

'I don't have schizophrenia, either.' I was looking at nurse leech but everyone could hear.

Guy and the nurse looked at me then turned away to continue their conversation. I knew they were ignoring me.

'I just couldn't sleep, for eighteen days. How would you feel if you hadn't slept for that long? You'd be off with the pixies, wouldn't you?' I wanted to bang my head on the punching bag that was hanging in the corner, to emphasise the futility of my situation.

'The sleeping tablets weren't working, the temazepam. They're addictive, aren't they? They lose their potency, don't they? I had to keep on increasing the amount.'

'Okay, Gardenia, I'm dealing with Guy's problems first. Perhaps you could find your nurse and talk to her?'

'About which came first, the chicken or the egg? Do you know?' I said.

'No, but I don't think it's just the temazepam that has caused your illness,' said the male nurse.

'Or not sleeping for eighteen days?' I said.

'I grant you it would have an impact,' said the nurse. His quiet demeanour made me feel like throwing him in the fountain.

'Then it would make me psychotic?'

'Yes, it could.'

'Thank you for a direct answer.' I felt like I had won the battle of wits.

'A person suffering with the diagnosis of depression or psychosis can be related to a person who is paraplegic, or quadriplegic. The debilitating effect and distress is just as serious,' the nurse said.

'And that's supposed to make me feel better?' I wished I had not started the conversation.

'I can understand why you're angry, Gardenia. I think that will be enough for one day,' the nurse said.

'You can say that again,' I said.

'Do you know that we all lie,' Guy said. 'If I said "How are you?", what would you answer?'

I wondered if it was some kind of trick question.

'I would say how I've been feeling,' said the nurse. 'Talk about my visits to the doctor or my depression.'

'Do you have depression?' the girl said.

'Really?' said Guy. 'But you wouldn't say that to a person you don't know?'

'No, I would just say I'm all right,' the nurse continued.

'Then that would be a lie, if you weren't feeling all right.'

'Yes, you have a point, Guy,' said the nurse. His beady eyes were getting smaller. I wondered if he felt threatened.

'You can't tell a person working at the supermarket checkout that you just found out you had terminal cancer or your cat just died and by the way I'm on tablets because my doctor thinks I'm psychotic,' Guy said. He smiled as if he had just won Mastermind.

'It has to be proper, like, doesn't it?' said the girl.

I had a vision of sitting in the back garden of a huge mansion in Devon, England, drinking cups of tea from Royal Doulton cups and eating cucumber sandwiches.

The nurse turned to Guy. 'I'll see what your notes say. I can probably give you something to help your anxiety.' He stood up and turned to open the door. He walked away and Guy followed him.

He's probably going to give him his mid-morning medication, a mild sedative.

'I'll see you later then, girls, and remember we don't know what the future holds.' Guy waved and smiled.

I didn't want to get on the wrong side of this authoritarian structure. I knew the consequences – to be locked in a secure ward, or sedated. I thought about prison and how inmates bribed or coerced others to get what they wanted. I didn't want to submit to corrupt prison officers. I had principles. *Am I being paranoid? They could keep me here, just for being opinionated.*

I felt like throwing something, anything. I wanted to pick up the ashtrays and hurl them into the fountain. I decided against it. I didn't want to be in this prison hospital longer than was necessary.

'By the way, can you smell something burning?' the younger girl said.

'No. What do you mean? Is this place on fire?' I said.

'No, it's just that the doctor asked me that before. He said that if you can smell something like burning, it means you have schizophrenia,' she said.

'Too bad if you smoke cigarettes – you could be locked up for good,' I said.

The girl laughed.

'I'm exhausted, I'm going to bed,' I said.

'It's a bit early, isn't it? You're not going to leave me here alone, are you?'

I looked at her. I wanted to say something nice, helpful, but I couldn't think of a thing to say.

I returned to my room. I couldn't lie down on my bed for long. I felt restless. I thought about getting a soft drink and then talking to a nurse to have a deep meaningful conversation. The drink machine was outside in another area next to the dining room. A can of Coke would make things better, like the advertising slogan. Maybe wake me up and change me into an energetic fun-loving slim bimbo.

Hardly.

I passed some nurses and said 'Hello', smiling at them pleasantly. I was too afraid to say anything that wasn't appropriate.

An obese nurse passed me as I slipped the coins into the machine.

'You shouldn't drink that rubbish, especially that Coke,' she said. 'You won't sleep tonight if you drink that all day.'

I wanted to say I had been without sleep for several days and it wasn't due to the Coca Cola, but to doctors giving me addictive sleeping tablets, but I was scared of the backlash.

'It isn't good for you,' she continued.

Yes, it increases your weight. So you better not have any because you won't fit through the doorway soon. Should I say it? I looked at my ever-expanding stomach. *I can't tell her she's fat, it isn't polite. Mind you, they're telling me I'm insane. I wonder if she's in a bad mood. If she isn't, then I'm in trouble.*

I acquiesced to her judgement and nodded. I changed my preference to Fanta instead. *Why do they have the machine here in the first place?*

I waited for the machine to do its mechanical movement and it didn't. *It's obviously malfunctioning. Perhaps if I use my telepathic powers, a can will pop out.*

Suddenly the machine worked. *That's a bit scary,* I thought.

I knew any inappropriate comments would be noted, saying I was uncooperative or abusive. If I appeared happy, I was sure they would diagnose me with a mood disorder. *Can Fanta make you manic?*

I walked to the nurses' station and sat down near the foyer, hoping to attract someone's attention. I waited, watching the nurses and patients go by. I hoped a nurse would notice me. When fifteen minutes had ticked by, I decided it was time to assert my rights.

'Excuse me,' I said to a nurse passing by. 'I want to talk to someone.'

'Sure,' the young female nurse replied. 'Who is your nurse today?'

'I have no idea.'

'I'll have a look for you then.' She went back to the nurses' station and looked up on the notice board. 'It's Cordelia,' she said. 'She's having her break. She won't be long. I'll let her know you're waiting.'

I watched the clock on the wall impatiently as thirty minutes ticked by. I looked at the Van Gogh print on the wall, the blue irises. They seemed to be moving. I wondered if it was a hallucination, or I was just tired. I was getting sick of waiting, but then I wasn't in a hurry to go anywhere.

'Excuse me,' I said to another nurse passing by. 'I've been told Cordelia's my nurse today. I've been waiting for ages. Can you help me?'

'You want to speak to Cordelia?'

'Yes.'

'Okay, I'll go and find her. She's around somewhere.'

I waited for what seemed another thirty minutes. Just as I was going to give up, Cordelia appeared, smiling and excusing herself for being so long.

'Sorry, Gardenia, I had some urgent business.'

It must be a difficult job. Probably like being in an emergency ward? The patients are quite collected. I don't think they're hanging themselves in a quiet place somewhere. I haven't seen anyone running around screaming. At least, I don't think so. How do the nurses know what's wrong with a person's mind? Is it just instinct or are they trained to assume people are mad in general? I suppose experience gives them some foundation.

'How are you? Would you like to talk?'

Cordelia looked like a wannabe Marilyn Monroe. She had everything going for her – the platinum-blonde hair, the sleek small nose. Blue doe eyes that looked sympathetic. I wondered about her nature, if she would be nice. I presumed there would be a flaw.

I nodded.

'Come into one of the consulting rooms.'

I sat opposite Cordelia and looked at my pink sandshoes, avoiding eye contact. 'I feel like I can't cope. That's an understatement. I'm scared, all the time, especially of people and going out. Sometimes I feel like everything will explode in my mind. I'll die in torture, a horrible and painful death. Or my life will continue and I'll live an excruciating senseless existence.' I felt like my words would never stop. It was only with a sheer act of will that I stopped myself talking in tongues. I was sure I got the point across. But that was only the tip of the iceberg.

'I understand,' Cordelia said.

'I feel like I'm a leper.' I felt like throwing up. I wanted to stop thinking this way, to try and relax, but that made it worse. I was panicking and I gulped in some air.

'Perhaps you're just thinking this way now,' said Cordelia.

'I could think differently about the situation, you mean? If I decide to think hopelessly about things, then obviously I'll feel hopeless.' I wanted this construct to be true. 'I do have some hope, you know.' Tears were starting to drip down my cheek.

Cordelia reached over and gave me a tissue.

I blew heavily from my nose. 'Thank you,' I said. 'This mental health system, they won't hurt me, will they?' I continued. 'I'm not mad and I'm not weird. I've been trying for years to make you and others believe that.'

Cordelia listened. She was watching me try to express myself. My hands were moving wildly about in the air. I wondered if the nurse could really help. It was like having faith in the unknown. It was usually while I was in this state of fear that any help was an improbability.

'It's comforting to realise that you have a mental illness. At least there's a reason why you feel this way. To receive help medically and know what you're dealing with is part way in finding the solution,' Cordelia said.

I know that!

'Yeah, but everything is horrible.'

'I think life is hard for a great deal of people. How you look at life will help you. There are many roads to recovery.'

Oh God, how philosophical, but is it practical?

'Are you troubled about going home?' Cordelia said.

Why do all the nurses talk about living arrangements? Guy had problems at home.

'Yes, I don't know, maybe. I have no one to turn to, only my mother. She's getting older and she's tired. Mum usually does the shopping, pays the bills and everything.' I thought I was sounding selfish. 'How will I manage with all the financial stuff when she's gone?' The thought made me terrified. *Poor Cordelia, she has to listen to all these complaints every day.*

'Perhaps you can talk to your doctor about seeing a social worker. There are also community nurses. There's a lot of help out there, caring for the disabled.'

Does this nurse really understand my situation? I'm not bloody disabled.

'When you're feeling better, things will look different. Your doctor has you on some new antidepressants. Wait until they've worked and then think about these issues.'

I hope she's right. At least she's being positive. I thought about the electric shock treatment and the idea of short-term memory loss. That would cause anxiety, not being able to remember what you just thought about. *Perhaps that's why I can't concentrate.*

'I know ECT can make you lose your memory, but does it come back?' I knew the question sounded stupid. Can you function at all without a memory?

'Yes, your memory does come back,' Cordelia said.

'How long does it take?'

'It should return within six months.'

I appreciated the honest answer.

I thought about the ECT treatment at Felixstowe. I had lost count of the number of times I had been strapped down. If I was so withdrawn and I knew I was not well, then that might have been the cause. That's why they thought I had a psychotic problem? I had no way of going back to tell the doctors otherwise.

'I might sit in the garden for a while, try and get some vitamin D,' I said.

'That's a good idea. I'll write in your notes that you wish to see a social worker too.'

Why do I need to see a social worker? I felt the cogs in my brain trying to work. I needed some grease to push them along. I was talking about my mother wasn't I, and about finance? Yes, that was it.

I followed the nurse from the consulting room and walked through the corridors, past other patients and nurses. I was not quite familiar yet with the plan of the hospital and recognising faces.

In the garden, I saw Guy and Libby again and I sat down next to them.

'I find the drugs make you less aware. Like you can't feel anything,' Guy said.

I understood his dilemma. I would never be able to decipher medicine and its effects.

'I've got bipolar,' Guy said.

Libby and I didn't respond. The term didn't give any meaning. I only thought it meant high and low moods, which was a simple assumption.

'I mean, I try all this therapy and it doesn't work. I end up pretending all this stuff to try and make myself feel better. Why do I have to accept an illness when the doctors don't know the half of it?'

I knew what Guy was talking about, but I didn't want to reflect on his problems.

An elderly man came out to the patio area. He sat down next to me. He had a long straggly beard and resembled a castaway who had been living alone on an island. 'I'm not like you,' he said. 'You're in space and flying but you're not attached to anything. You're a lost soul, a spirit that can never be real. You're dead and you're going to keep on going around and round in space always lost, dead in hell.'

Well, that's a great way of opening a conversation. How dare he call me a lost spirit?

'Yes, you're going to hell, you'll never be at peace,' the old man said.

Obviously he's sick, but I shouldn't have to put up with this sort of abuse. I thought that his ideas weren't far from the truth. This place was a living hell.

Suddenly a noise like a loud alarm clock rang out.

'It's the bloody fire alarm again, probably just a routine thing,' said Guy.

I looked at the sign on the brick pillar that was in front of me. It stated 'Red spot area for emergency'.

'Do we have to gather here in case of fire?' I said.

'Well, that means we're safe here, doesn't it?' said Guy. He moved closer to the brick pillar.

'Fire,' the old man yelled. 'We're going to fry in hell. We'll be lost spirits, forever.'

'We're outside and we can leave by that gate, if we have to. We're not in danger,' said Libby.

I felt myself shaking but my body was rigid at the same time. I thought I was going to involuntarily jump like a cork out of a bottle. I picked up my coffee cup, trying to disguise my shaking hand. *If I pretend I'm just doing a normal everyday thing, my panic attack or whatever it is will go away.* This only made my anxiety increase and my arm jerked and I threw the coffee mug all over the old man sitting next to me.

'Why did you do that?' he said. His eyes were big and blue. They reminded me of the marbles I used to play with as a child.

'I'm sorry,' I said. 'I couldn't help it. I feel hot,' I continued. 'I don't think I'm perspiring. Shouldn't I be sweating in this heat?'

'It's the antipsychotics,' said Libby. 'They stop your sweat glands from working. I've heard there have been fatalities. It's best to sit in the shade.'

I looked at Libby and wondered if she was right.

Libby had read my mind. 'Yes, it's true, I tell you. I don't know why, but it happens,' she said.

People exaggerate their medical conditions all the time, but I was not going to doubt Libby's sincerity. She looked like she had seen it all.

Now I'm supposed to be some night creature. Next I'll be sucking blood.

'I like your slippers, they're fluffy and cute and they look like smiling cats. They're alive, though, aren't they, not dead like you?' the old man said.

I looked at my pink sandshoes. I couldn't see the resemblance. 'I don't like you saying my cat slippers are dead.' I was trying very hard to handle the conversation and to be objective.

'They're going to be with you in a lost world, when you're dead. They're going to guide you into hell. That's why the Egyptians put them in their tombs.'

'Why? So they could go to hell?' I said and looked at Libby and frowned. 'If he keeps on with this dead stuff, I'm going to really yell at him. He'll be living in a lost world in a minute,' I said.

'The sky is blue but then spiders are like glue and if your face is wet or your limitations aren't met, then you've a chance to go to the loo,' the old man said.

Is that meant to be funny? You could hang that poem on the back of a toilet door. What does he mean by not having your limitations met? Can you exceed your limitations? Do you want to be limited? Is your work not good enough? That would mean not having your expectations met?

I felt like asking him what he meant but knew he'd quickly created the words. He hadn't written a thesis on it.

Suddenly I realised what he meant. He wanted to say he was a horrible ugly person who was devoid of all reason.

The old man blew his nose loudly. I looked at him to see if he had a hanky. He didn't.

Libby fossicked around in her purse and gave him a used tissue. 'Well, it's better than nothing,' she said.

'These things can be utilised for lots of things. Not just as a nose-blowing material,' said the old man, looking at his tissue.

I didn't want to ask him what else they could be used for.

The ringing siren of a fire engine could be heard in the distance.

'Everyone stay focused,' said Libby.

'The nurse will be here soon, I think,' said Guy.

'I was in Vietnam,' said the old man.

'Oh yes, and you'll fight the fire then?' I said.

'Just calm down,' said Libby.

The gardener came in through the wooden gate. He was ready to start his work for the day. He pulled his hose and garden equipment behind him.

'Quick, let's make our escape,' Guy said.

That gate was open all the time. We're just a bunch of losers.

I watched the gardener standing looking at a plant. Then he went back outside of the hospital leaving the gate wide open. He returned and looked at the plant again and then walked out through the gate once more.

I'm not the only one suffering from memory loss. I thought of running away. *They'll eventually find me and bring me back. Probably detain me. There really isn't any point, other than the exercise.*

'I bet this old man has pulled some cord or pressed some button, probably the fire alarm. Why do we have to stand here next to this brick pole? Is it going to save us?' I said.

'My name is John,' said the old man.

A nurse came through the double glass doors. She was a small blonde young woman. She assessed the situation. 'Everyone okay?' she said.

'Yes, except for him, he's really lost his marbles,' I said. 'Why do we have to put up with his complete nonsense?'

'Everyone's sick,' Libby said.

'Yes, and he's really sick.'

'What's going on, Gardenia? Perhaps we should have a talk?' said the nurse.

'He's the one who needs therapy,' I said and pointed to John. 'I'm sorry. I just can't deal with this at the moment. I don't want to die and be a lost spirit forever dangling in the sky. He's making me scared. He told me that my furry slippers were going to take me to hell, like in Egyptian mummy tombs.'

'Did you?' the nurse looked at John and then at Gardenia's feet.

'We're all sick here. John is very sick, obviously, and Gardenia is suffering from something. No one means to say what they do. We just all have to understand each other's needs,' Libby said.

'Well that's sorted out then,' said the nurse. Her mobile phone rang. She pressed a button and put it to her ear. 'Yes, yes, okay.' She pushed another button and looked at the small group. 'It's finished, the firemen have assessed the situation. They've located the fire, which wasn't a fire, thank God.'

'What was it then? A planned attack or drill, just to scare us?' I said.

'It was someone spraying an aerosol can into the smoke alarm. Someone used a deodorant sanitiser in their bathroom. It must have triggered the alarm system,' said the nurse.

'Did they mean to do it?' I said.

'I don't think so,' said the nurse.

'Does it matter?' said Libby.

'What happens if they do it again?' I asked.

'They won't,' said the nurse.

'How do you know?' I looked at John.

'I don't know but I've been told that the person in question won't do it again,' said the nurse.

'You're making that up.'

'No, I'm not, Gardenia. I just think you need to stay calm.'

'Calm! Have a look at John. You can't tell me he won't do something stupid? I wouldn't be surprised if he climbs that ladder there and goes to that air-conditioning hub thing and blows us all up. See, they even have a ladder. What are they doing with a ladder there? What happens if someone tries to commit suicide, right in front of us?'

'You're catastrophising, Gardenia,' said the nurse.

'How much does it cost to send a fire engine here every five minutes? No wonder private health insurance is expensive,' I said.

'That's not very far from the ground, that ladder. If anyone jumps, they certainly wouldn't hurt themselves,' said Libby.

'I think we're all getting a bit overwhelmed. The probability of anyone jumping is a very low risk,' said the nurse.

'You mean to say that John is low risk and is not capable of setting the place alight, probably thinking we're all evil spirits and should be condemned to purgatory? He's capable of anything. Even talking about this could give him the idea to go and do it. He's making my life hell. Tell him to go away, he's weird. I just want a peaceful life, is that too much to ask? Anyway, he's probably a dirty old man. I've been molested before, you know.'

'Okay, Gardenia, we'll go inside. You can take your medication, prn, it will calm you down. Also your doctor is here.'

'What does prn stand for again?' I said.

'It's medication that's prescribed when necessary,' said the nurse.

'Yes, just give me the drugs and everything will be okay?'

I followed the nurse into the hospital. I looked at John and poked my tongue out. I went to the nurses' station and was given a small blue pill. I then waited for my doctor outside the consulting rooms, near the nurses' station. I checked my watch. I was intent on going home. It was only a case of winning the doctor over and saying that the antidepressants had kicked in. It might not work, but there was no harm in trying.

4

I saw my doctor arrive. She was laughing and joking with the nurses.

What's she got to laugh about? Why is anyone happy?

Doctor Jarvie walked towards me. She looked elegant in her printed shirt. The autumn leaf pattern coordinated with her light brown skirt. I looked at her shoes and they were a light camel colour.

'Hello, Gardenia. Let's see if this room is vacant, shall we?'

Where else can we go? She's supposed to be clever and I've got my life in her hands. I hope she knows what she's doing.

Doctor Jarvie didn't sit at the desk but in one of the comfortable armchairs. I sat opposite her. I watched her looking through my ever-expanding file. She scribbled some notes. I wanted to ask if I could see her notes. I decided against it. I didn't want to know.

'How are you going with the alprazolam?'

'I think it's helping.'

Doctor Jarvie was not threatening, but gentle in her approach. I couldn't help feeling better. I looked at the room, its immaculate appearance. The clean, freshly painted walls. Restful colours dominated the hospital's décor with pastel hues and touches of saturated pigment. *I could study colour theory in this hospital. Colour coordination is a fashionable trend.*

'Good.' The doctor wrote some more notes. 'Your mother has been a great support, hasn't she?'

'She has gone through hell.'

'It's not your fault. I'm sorry for how the medical system has treated you.'

She keeps on saying that. I wonder what she means.

'I can't urinate because I'm so scared,' I said. I thought I'd get to the point. I remembered having a catheter at Felixstowe and I didn't want to go through that again.

'That might be the medication – it causes fluid retention. It might be a muscular problem. The nurse can give you something for that.'

So it's not my fault? I'd been under the impression that because I was so neurotic or stark raving mad it was my problem. Now she's saying it's the medication. That's a relief.

'What medication causes that?' I asked.

'Some minor tranquillisers can have such an effect,' she said.

I wonder if she's just saying that. It may be her way of trying to lessen my anxiety? They have their methods.

'Has your depression lifted?'

'Everything looks brighter.' I was getting used to the nice environment. It reminded me of an expensive health resort. I wasn't delusional. It was still a mental hospital.

The doctor wrote down some more notes.

'I don't want to be in hospital.'

'That's a healthy sign. These hospitals used to be called asylums, meaning places of refuge.'

I wish other people could see it like that.

'Like asylum seekers who come on boats trying to have a better life?' I thought it better to agree with the doctor's theories. I knew I was feeling sorry for myself. People were dying every minute. Some had nothing, no money, nothing to eat and children were dying of leukaemia every day. It didn't make me feel better about myself, comparing my life with those who were worse off. Rather, it made me confused that life had to be such a sad struggle.

'I don't want to be categorised or judged.'

'No one's judging you, Gardenia. You're free to come and go as you like. We're only here to help you, not to cast judgement, or even to give your problem a name.'

'Am I detained?'

'No, but we have to know where you go, just for safety reasons. I've been thinking that respite would be beneficial. You would learn some independent living skills and your mother would have a break.'

I didn't like this idea.

'You'd be living in a community house. It's part of a government rehabilitation scheme and private health companies are helping with the financial costs. Social interaction programmes on managing mental illness are part of the project. Your mother would get help from community services with shopping and cleaning. Here, I have a brochure. Perhaps think about it, Gardenia.'

I took the brochure. I was not interested in the slightest.

'Can lack of sleep cause hallucinations?' I asked. 'I haven't experienced anything like voices before.'

'Are you still having them?'

'No, they've gone, I think.' I waited for a moment to hear the usual sarcasm of some ethereal being. 'Do you think I have schizophrenia, Doctor Jarvie?'

'You can call me Alice.'

Really?

'No, I don't think I really understand the cause. You may have gone through an identity crisis.'

'I think I lost my identity. I had a termination, seven years ago. Everything went downhill from there. Mind you, things weren't going too well beforehand.'

'If it's any consolation, I do believe you when you say you've never experienced hallucinations before,' said Alice.

'I think I would have remembered. It was horrible.' *But then most people would give their right eye to talk to Jesus.* 'I was depressed at Felixstowe. I didn't like it there, so I ran home. They locked me up because of that.'

'I think they were wrong to do that. I'll keep you on the same medication. I'll lower the risperdal. I think the effexor can be increased a bit more and I think having you off the lithium will make you feel a lot better. I'll keep you on the alprazolam too. I also think it would be a good idea to take Epilem, as it'll help stabilise your moods.'

My mother had said beware of nice people and I realised she was right. Doctor Jarvie wasn't going to change anything. She was going to sit on the fence, play it safe and agree with the doctors at Felixstowe.

With that amount of medication in my system, I'll still be rattling like a walking medicine bottle. I still can't understand why I need all the tablets. I wanted to ask her, but I was tired of questioning my sanity. Explaining why I was okay, a good person. I just wanted someone to understand. I knew I couldn't afford to think negatively about Doctor Jarvie. I was in her hospital, so to speak, and she had power over my life, the control to do whatever she liked. I had seen enough security guards in mental hospitals to know this was true. If I stepped out of line for a moment, I'd be locked in a cell. *I wonder if they have prison quarters here in Kensington clinic. I'm seeing things negatively because she's trying to help me by decreasing some of the tablets. She said she was sorry on behalf of the system. Didn't she say I was over-medicated? At least she was honest about the tablets causing fluid retention.*

'Have you thought about going to the groups here? The programmes are run in the room just near the dining area. Have you looked at the leaflets in your room?'

'No, I didn't think this hospital had groups. I was told they have meetings but I haven't been to one.'

'The meetings are in the morning and the nurses inform you about the daily activities. You might like to join the other groups. Different subjects come up, like dealing with depression, and CBT classes are also held. I'll see you tomorrow night and perhaps we'll talk more about some rehabilitation, but we'll make you feel better first.'

I left the doctor and sat outside in the garden area again, under the porch. My memory told me that gardens, birds and bees, flowers and trees gave a person solace, peace. However, it didn't stop the menacing thoughts, the incongruities and my attempts to understand the reason for my circumstances.

I couldn't deny my existence. How could one forget the past? My fears were with me every moment, like a shadow, a dark strange concept that was illusive, but its impact was powerful and very real. I couldn't say when or how or why I was clinically diagnosed with a schizo-affective disorder. I could only understand the circumstances, the events and how I felt. These were the only factors that could connect me with a reality that had so far been incomprehensible. I had told Doctor Jarvie about the termination. Perhaps that was the reason, the cause. After all, it had happened just before my first admission. Like a spider's web, I tried to make connections that would strengthen my mind. To alleviate the discomfort of thinking myself mad. My only weapon was to go back to remember how it all began...

5

Felixstowe was a large public psychiatric hospital situated in the middle of Melbourne. I had never been inside the grounds before but I had seen the main building from a distance. I had always viewed it with a sense of fear.

As my mother and I slowly walked up the gravelled path, I noticed the building's elaborate colonial beauty. The front facades were artistic, with meticulous sculptured ironwork and stone masonry. A bougainvillea vine was crawling and sprawling within and around the columns and balconies.

I could imagine the interior of this structure. It would have a main reception room with a wide staircase leading to who knows where? All the rooms would be colossal, with high ceilings. The walls would be decorated with intricate tapestries depicting England in its former days or wealthy people sitting on thrones of some sort, looking down on the serfs. There would probably be framed ornate inscriptions revealing the building's historical details. It looked like an important sacred site. I felt small and insignificant as it towered above me.

I knew Felixstowe was financed by the government and patients who accessed the facility would have to be in the lower income bracket – those who couldn't afford private health insurance. I realised it would have to accommodate a lot of people, because who could afford hospital insurance these days – only the wealthy? *But then do people go to Felixstowe every day?*

I thought it was an institution and patients had to stay there. It wasn't like a general hospital, with surgery, and when recovered you were discharged. Wasn't it the custom that only serious medical cases were admitted – 'inmates' who had chronic conditions and deemed unfit to live in the wider community?

I heard a roar that sounded similar to waves beating on the shore in a storm. A car passed us as it drove down towards a parking bay. I heard the crunching of its tyres. My hearing was so sensitive – I was acutely aware of every noise. This aggravation made my head ache. I tried to keep out the stimuli of my surroundings but I couldn't close my eyes or stop my ears from working. I noticed the shiny reflections on the vehicles in the car park – the sleek sports cars, BMWs and other prestigious, expensive motors. I knew they were probably owned by the specialists. After all, would mental patients have that much money?

The first building had a sign on the front saying 'Reception'. It was a large red-brick modern structure with a hard-featured appearance. It did not have the elegance of the main building. It had a bleak and forbidding countenance. There were people huddled outside the front entrance. I wondered if they were dangerous to themselves or others.

'Don't be afraid of us,' a man said. 'We just roam around the place. We stick to the entrance ways, for our own protection.' He let out a scream and placed his hands around his throat.

I walked past the group, averting my eyes from their troubled, staring faces.

'Is it true that you're going to save us?' another of the men said.

'Yes, I'll sort it out,' I answered. *What else could I say?*

'Humanity is going to be saved,' the man sang out.

'Be careful, they're revolving doors,' another man said.

It was distressing. I could see they were tormented in one way or another – condemned to live in mental anguish. I couldn't become accustomed to this place. *Who would want to work here let alone live here?*

We came to the entrance way and the automatic sliding doors opened. I followed my mother into a large room. I noticed the grey walls and the grey carpeted floor. The white plastic chairs that sat in front of a glass cubicle. *Obviously the office.*

The simplicity of the modern furniture was artless. The designs and architectural influence of the interior had a single-minded purpose – functional. It was a whitewash of monotones, cleanliness and order. I watched my mother go to the counter and enquire about our appointment. The nurses in their white uniforms looked austere and cold.

They don't look very happy. Probably just waiting for their pay packet at the end of the week.

'Excuse me, I rang earlier because my daughter needs to see a doctor. We were told to come in, for a consultation.'

'You made an appointment?' said the nurse.

'Yes, they said to come in immediately,' my mother said.

'But that isn't an appointment, is it?'

'Yes, eleven-thirty. That was the time.' My mother was still pleasantly spoken even if the nurse wasn't.

'Okay, just take a seat and I'll see who is available.'

The waiting area consisted of eight chairs, four of them facing each other with a large coffee table with magazines piled in the middle. The chairs were plastic and uncomfortable and two men sat opposite me. Patients, I presumed, and they were staring at me.

I wondered how mentally ill they were. I knew they were only interested in one thing – probably sex offenders, I thought. I didn't want to imagine what they were thinking – what mad ideas and thoughts were going through their minds. I saw another young girl sitting with an older woman. She looked as miserable as I felt. My mind and body felt like a piece of wobbly jelly. I could literally feel my body trembling both internally and externally. The strain was difficult to bear – I felt vulnerable and acutely aware of my circumstances and I didn't like it.

We waited for what seemed hours, until a large-framed woman who had trouble breathing told me to follow her. I wondered if she had some form of emphysema. But more likely it was her weight that was causing her discomfort. I didn't have to look at my own trembling skinny fingers to know I was far too thin. I looked back at my mother and she smiled at me. It was comforting to know she would be there when I returned.

I followed the large figure through a doorway and down a hallway to another door.

'You can sit here and wait for the doctor.' She left and I wondered what sort of doctor it would be; perhaps a psychologist.

The room was bare with a desk and a chair for the doctor obviously and another chair that was situated at right angles to the desk. I had not waited long before a young man, casually dressed in a cotton T-shirt and brown cord pants, entered the room. He had dark hair and was wearing glasses.

'I'm Doctor Grimshaw,' he said. He sat down and placed a manila folder on the desk. He opened the file. 'You are Gardenia Baxter?' He didn't smile and his intense stare made me feel uncomfortable. He then looked at the papers in front of him.

'Yes.' I did know who I was in the literal sense.

'You're here because...?' He didn't finish the question. Doctor Grimshaw looked at his watch and he was waiting for me to speak.

I wanted to voice my distress but I couldn't find the right words.

'Your mother rang telling us you weren't feeling well. What seems to be the trouble?'

The room had a large window and I could see the foliage of a eucalypt tree and in the distance the city buildings.

'I haven't been feeling like myself,' I said.

'I see, and what makes you say that?'

I wondered how old he was. He looked only in his late twenties – if that. *Maybe he's a student doctor but they wouldn't have him making decisions about a person's life, would they?*

'You're twenty years of age – is that right?' he asked.

I nodded. *Did I answer his last question? My memory isn't very good.*

'I don't know what's wrong with me. I've had a rough time and I think I'm depressed,' I continued.

'Why is that?'

'I just had an abortion.'

I watched him writing down some notes.

'I was at university and I felt inferior and perhaps it was my fault that it happened. I must be making my mother distressed.'

'Have you had periods of depression before?'

'No, not really – only just hormone levels with premenstrual tension. I know I'm confused and I'm frightened and I can't concentrate. Sometimes it feels like déjà vu.'

'What are you frightened of?'

'I don't know. I was drinking heavily and taking drugs.'

'Yes, and what type of drugs?'

'Magic mushrooms, LSD, speed, marijuana.' I felt stupid. Lots of people take drugs and are not in mental hospitals. 'I'm sure it's all because of the termination.' *Didn't I just say that? I'm repeating myself.*

The doctor kept scribbling down his notes. 'And how is that making you feel now?'

Didn't he just ask that question? Isn't he supposed to know the effects of trauma? How else can I explain myself?

'I feel very shaky – teary, I suppose. I feel depressed and a bit unreal.'

'Unreal?' he said.

I saw his black eyebrows arch and I sensed danger. He intimidated me and I felt like some sort of test case.

'What does this unreal feeling make you think of? Can you describe it?'

I wasn't sure if he meant me to understand my problem. To describe it would mean I already knew the answers. Didn't they make the diagnoses? I started to wonder what his motives were and why he asked me for the answers.

'Have you been hearing voices – seeing things, anything unreal like that?'

It was then that I wished I had not said the word 'unreal'. I tried to discount my fears of being locked up indefinitely. That's what they do to people who are insane, who have hallucinations. I knew I was being investigated. I tried to control myself, my words.

'I've had problems recently with an ex-boyfriend and I've had drugs before in the past.' I was trying to explain the reasons for my being there, a plausible explanation for my confusion.

The doctor continued writing his notes.

'I can't understand the meaning of words.' I couldn't help myself from being honest. I knew I had said something that would get me into trouble.

He looked at me again and I was sure his eyes lit up as if he had just understood some mysterious secret or made a new discovery. I didn't like him or his attitude. I felt like a piece of meat – a frightened animal cornered. He was pursuing me like a hunter and he had the advantage. I was in his lair and he knew he had the power. I only hoped he had the intelligence to use this power with wisdom, compassion.

'What are your anxieties?'

'I feel fearful in crowds, and I can't socialise. I live a withdrawn lifestyle.' These general questions were irritating me.

'You don't know why you're agitated?'

Didn't I just say what I'd been through?

I realised then that he was questioning my sanity.

'It's probably the termination – I'll be all right. I'm not guilty.' I didn't like this kind of analyses. I shifted my feet and I felt goosebumps crawling on my skin.

'What are your thoughts?'

'My thoughts? I don't understand.' I felt his eyes boring into me and I looked out of the window, pretending I wasn't frightened. 'I can see a tree out there and birds flying.' *Is that what he means by a thought?*

'Your development – was it normal, with school friends?'

'Yes, I was very good at school with top marks and then university. I was a prefect too.' I felt like I was being judged and had to prove my adequacy.

'And how do you get on with your mother?'

'My mum and I get on really well.'

'Always?'

What does he mean by that?

'When did you have your first sexual experience and how did you feel about it?'

I did not like his ideas or the inquisition and where this conversation was going.

'I don't really enjoy sex. The person has to be right so that I can feel okay about it.' *I am not going to disclose any more information. I'll just let him know I haven't been feeling well but I'll be all right.*

'I'm just not sleeping well and I'm a bit worried about my health. I'll be better soon, thank you. Well, I can't say there are fairies down the bottom of the garden, can I?' I tried to make a joke but it didn't have any effect. It didn't make me feel any better and he certainly didn't see the humour. *I wonder if he does think I see fairies at the bottom of the garden?*

'I think it's in your best interests to take the medication I'm going to prescribe and also you need to be admitted just for a week. We need to do some tests – just to see what's going on.' He smiled.

It was the first time I had noticed his teeth. They were jagged like stalagmites. Spear-like protrusions that you would normally find in dark caves. I wondered if he was happy to have made this decision. Did he enjoy admitting patients, or in some macabre way was he trying to make me feel better?

'I think it should happen immediately. Is that your mother waiting out there?'

I nodded. I wanted to leave, to say it was okay, but I was too tired to fight.

He got up and I followed him back into the main reception area. My mother was still there waiting.

'Mrs Baxter? I'm Doctor Grimshaw. I think as I have just told Gardenia that she should be admitted – just for a short time.'

'Mum, everything's all right. I don't need to stay here.'

'I think it's in her best interests, Mrs Baxter,' he said and I could see the stalagmites again.

'We have some medication that will make her feel better but we have to know her situation.'

What am I looking for? A place to rent?

'I see.' My mother was agreeing with him – I couldn't believe it.

'Can you bring back her clothes, toiletries, concession cards and all that and we'll admit her now. Okay?'

'This is all a bit sudden. I don't think it's necessary, is it, Gardenia?'

'No, it isn't,' I said. I was relieved to know my mother was questioning his authority.

'I think you'll be finding that at home Gardenia will not get better.'

Why isn't he talking to me? I looked at my mother pleadingly. I could see she was worried.

'Yes, I wouldn't want her to get worse. I do want her to have some help.'

No, Mum, don't do it, don't agree to this!

'Well, this is the best place,' he said.

I don't think so.

'Gardenia, perhaps we'll go across to the shopping centre and get something to eat.'

I thought that my mother had understood me. That she knew I didn't want to be hospitalised. I was glad to walk back up the gravelled driveway and out of the gates. It seemed to me that once we had eaten we would be making our way home. Instead, my mother took me to the nearest department store, saying how I needed new pyjamas. I wondered why she wanted to buy me the dressing gown too and the slippers, but I did appreciate her kindness. Perhaps it was gift to make me feel better? I didn't want to contemplate the real reason. I took the parcels in my arms, ready to take the taxi cab home.

'I suppose we should be getting back,' she said.

'Home?' I answered.

'No, we're going back to the hospital.'

I felt weak, like I was going to faint. 'You don't mean that, surely, Mum?'

'The doctor said it was the best thing for you, Gardenia. It won't be for long and you'll be feeling much better.'

I knew that it was not that simple but I wanted to believe her.

My mother left me to walk back to the hospital while she took a taxi home – she was going to pack a suitcase for me.

'You will go back there, Gardenia. Please trust me,' she said.

I looked at her and nodded. Then I turned away from her and walked back. I didn't see the patients huddled around the entrance again, thank God. I wasn't sure what to do or where to go, so I sat in the reception area, on the white plastic seat and waited. I saw Doctor Grimshaw talking to the nurses.

'Did you have a good holiday?' one nurse asked.

'Oh yes, I loved Spain. You must go, you know. It's really worth it,' Doctor Grimshaw replied.

The young nurse smiled. The doctor didn't see me sitting in the waiting area.

'Gardenia Baxter is going to be admitted, this afternoon. She doesn't want to come in and I am afraid she'll be an absconding risk. Make sure she's detained, won't you?'

'Yes, I'll make sure all the forms are correct. Don't worry,' said the nurse.

I saw Doctor Grimshaw leave. I bent my head down and cried silently. My mother was the only one I trusted on this earth and she wanted me to stay here. I felt she had abandoned me and I didn't understand why.

*

Felixstowe Hospital
Outpatient Record
Duty Doctor: G Grimshaw

Gardenia Baxter is a 20-year-old woman and is currently unemployed and lives with mother.
Referral: mother.
Gardenia is displaying confusion: 'I have lost the meaning of words'. Has poor concentration and memory and has difficulty in thinking through abstract ideas. She is neatly dressed 'trendy student style' and cooperative but has a flat blunted affect. Little rapport.
Has had a termination but doesn't feel guilty about it now.
Has disorientation and difficulty in thinking through abstract topics. Has problems trying to express her thoughts, ideas, feelings coherently.
Has confusion about her identity but not to gender or sexuality. Tearful episodes and some sadness; also

reports feelings of déjà vu.
On specific questioning there is no evidence of symptoms
of schizophrenia or overt psychosis.
No mood variation although has excessive guilt.
Recent drugs: marijuana and alcohol.
Precipitatory illnesses: none that she could identify.
Formal cognitive testing has not been done. There is
no evidence that she is floridly psychotic.

Diagnosis
Axis 1
Identity disorder of adolescence
Affective disorder - major
Adjustment disorder with depressed mood
Schizophrenic disorder
Organic mental disorder
Substance abuse disorder: cannabis, alcohol

Plan
Diagnostic admission
Needs full blood tests
Full physical examination
EEG
Mood, sleep, appetite chart
Complete history taking
Interview mother
Commencing fluphenazine 5 mg bd

Signed
Doctor G. Grimshaw

6

It wasn't long before the nurse, who had been speaking to Doctor Grimshaw, made her way across to me. I knew it was only a matter of time before someone would acknowledge me.

'Hello, Gardenia, I'm Wendy. We have to fill out some forms and I need your autograph,' she said. 'Can you come with me?'

I wanted to say of course I would be happy to follow you anywhere but refrained from making a sarcastic comment. I followed her into a large open area.

'This is the day room,' she said.

Lovely. Did you decorate it yourself?

It was an area larger than the size of my mother's home. I could see a pool table to one side and a lounge area. Then further towards the back of the unit was another lounge area with a television and another pool table. To the other side on the right was, I presumed, the dining area. The carpet was again grey and the brick walls were also painted grey. The couches and chairs were a somewhat different colour scheme – grey but with white flecks. I could see only a handful of other patients. One was spread out on a couch nearest the entrance. Another patient was sitting staring me at me as I entered and three other patients were watching television. I say patients because I presumed they weren't there for the fun and frivolity.

We sat down in the dining area.

'I have to have your particulars – name, address, birth date. Do you have your Medicare card and other health care cards?'

I nodded. At least I had enough sense to carry those things in my bag. I looked down to make sure I still had my backpack with me.

Wendy had a manila folder and forms inside. She quickly wrote the details of the cards down and I told her my full name, address, telephone number, date of birth. She was ticking boxes and writing notes. I hesitated to ask what she was writing, thinking it was only administrative details and therefore the content would be rudimentary. I was still making no headway in terms of communicating my thoughts to anyone, in relation to my admission and the reasons for it.

'Am I crazy?' I said. *Well, why not ask the obvious? A direct question certainly makes life easier, doesn't it?*

She looked at me and then continued writing.

I knew that I was going through some kind of bereavement process, but I had no idea what it entailed. I was in an unreal world but was hesitant to think that they could see me as someone experiencing some kind of schizophrenia. I mean, I had just told her who I was, my birth date. I had my health care cards.

She finished her writing and had me sign the papers. I did trust them to a degree and I didn't read the small writing on each of the papers, because I was just too tired to concentrate. I did forget about the doctor mentioning detainment – perhaps it was important for me to forget such a thing? My memory wasn't that wonderful – I just thought as a volunteer patient I would have the freedom to come and go as I pleased.

'I'm just a bit confused but I'm sure it's just a by-product of grief. You know, when someone close to you has died.' I wondered if she knew about the termination.

She looked at me again and I wondered if she was going to answer or make a comment about my circumstances?

'There will be a nurse along shortly to show you to your room. Okay?' With that remark, she got up and took her folder and walked towards the front entrance of the day room.

I have just killed a person. Don't you understand? The words echoed loudly in my mind.

I sat at the table for some time, just looking into space. *I'll just sit here and wait, soon it will be over and I'll be able to go back home.*

I noticed the red phone on the wall and wondered if I had to pay for the calls. I kept on looking towards the entrance watching for the arrival of my mother. *It's like waiting for a bus that isn't going to show up. Don't worry. It will be okay, everything will be all right.* I wondered why I even had to dispel such fear.

Another nurse arrived – she was an attractive woman, tall, dark-haired. 'I'm going to show you your room, okay?' she said.

I nodded and followed the nurse to the stairs. As we got closer to the top, I could hear someone screaming. It was a woman's voice. When we reached the first floor, I saw in front of me a door that had a small square window and through this glass I could see a woman's face. Her contorted features and her agonising pleas made me feel sick.

'Let me out. I won't do anything. Please let me out.'

I stared in horror, understanding the implications it meant for me – that I was in a hospital that locked people up. I staggered, wanting to turn and run quickly from the facility. As if the nurse read my thoughts, she pushed me towards another doorway.

'The woman – you have to let her out. She wants to get out,' I said.

The nurse's dark eyes looked straight through me as if I wasn't there. 'Don't worry about her, she's all right. This is your room.'

I looked at the doorknob wondering if it had a lock. Then I saw a bed and a chest of drawers beside it and a wardrobe that partitioned off the other bed in the room. I could still hear the girl screaming.

'When your mother brings your things, you can put them in there,' she said, pointing to the wardrobe door.

Well, where else would I put them?

'The showers are there across the room.' She pointed out of the doorway to another wall where there were more doors. 'Now, you have to come downstairs with me, because you're not allowed up here during the day, okay?'

Not during the day?

I followed her out of the room and down the hallway again. The sight of the poor woman had made me panic and I couldn't formulate an idea. My mind sensed impending doom. I wanted to leave the upstairs floor – I didn't want to acknowledge the fact that a woman was kept prisoner.

As we walked back down the corridor, the nurse pointed to another door. 'That's the TV room – you can only go in there after tea when you're ready for bed, okay. Got that?'

I nodded. I didn't particularly want to continue the conversation. We left each other at the bottom of the stairs.

'Tea is at five o'clock,' she said and briskly walked off.

When I saw my mother sitting in the lounge area, my relief was enormous. Even the appearance of the suitcase couldn't dispel my pleasure. I sat down next to my mother hoping that it was all a dreadful mistake and that we were going home.

'It's very nice here, isn't it?' she said.

I didn't know what to say.

'How have you settled in? Getting to know everyone?' she asked.

I wondered what planet she was on. 'I've just seen a woman locked up in a cell screaming to be let out,' I said. *If that doesn't make an impact, I don't know what will.*

'I don't think so, Gardenia, you're just making that up, you're not well. This is a nice place. I've brought you in some clothes. You just need a rest, that's all. I'm sure they're going to build you up with some vitamin B, that sort of thing.'

My conversation with my mother was increasing my frustration. My fears were escalating and culminating in what I thought was going to be some form of fit.

'The doctors are helping you. It's all just a preventative measure. Don't be frightened, Gardenia. Everything will be all right.'

My mother left just before teatime. She said she couldn't stay any longer because she had to feed the dog. *If only I was a dog. It couldn't be worse than being here. At least I could have a home, be fed, kept warm, given pats.*

I watched the patients move from their chairs in the lounge area, where they had been watching television. They marched towards the dining area. It was the first time I had seen so many people move at the same time.

They must be looking forward to it, I thought. It occurred to me that it was the only interesting thing in their day.

The dining area consisted of four long tables set out in a shape of a rectangle although separated by chairs in between. There was a long bench that was the serving area. It was not unlike a McDonalds where you went up and ordered your McHappy meal. I giggled at the irony as I watched the two women behind the counter. I must admit that hygiene rules were followed. They wore their hair up tied back under their hats. *Just as well.*

I didn't know what was on the menu. I saw the silver heating pans and saw the catering staff lift the tops off and reveal the peas and potatoes, their steam evaporating into the air. I saw the lasagne in another tub of stainless steel swimming in its tomato juices. I watched the patients one by one pick up a plate from the servery and state how much they wanted. I saw the custard rice cream at the end of the counter. That was all I wanted to eat.

The girl who had been screaming in the locked room was there. I couldn't mistake her face – I think it will be imprinted on my brain for the rest of my life. She was very bright, happy and talking.

She sat down opposite me. 'Don't worry. You'll be okay,' she said. She talked about her love of pottery and how she was going to have an exhibition.

It was as if nothing had happened. I wondered if it was a continuing situation for her – a daily routine and she was just so used to it, that it made little impact. I really didn't want to be social or talk niceties. Say 'Isn't the weather wonderful' or 'I like the food, don't you?' Nor did I want to talk at length about the reasons for insanity. I didn't have anything against these people, not personally. I just didn't want to be like them.

'You know we have a craft room here and you can paint miniature figurines,' she said.

I couldn't think of anything worse. *Do they think I'm retarded?*

'See that man there?' she said.

I looked at a man sitting across from me. He had dark hair – an Arabic appearance.

'Be wary of him, that's all I say,' she said. She curled her blonde hair around her finger – her eyes were a startling blue and seemed to have a life of their own.

Then a young man walked through the entrance and sat down at our table.

'Oh, hello, Jim,' she said.

He had long blond hair tied back in a ponytail. The top of his hair was cropped.

'Been out today, Glenda?' He looked at my reluctant compatriot.

'No. Did you want to go out?'

'I've already been out,' he replied.

'Oh yeah. What did you do?'

'Just some stuff to sort out.'

I looked from one to the other.

Isn't a conversation an exchange of ideas or thoughts? Is there a point to this drivel? I had not bargained for living with people who were obviously intellectually challenged. *This is a serious place – it has serious implications. Don't they understand that? What are they so happy about? Can you think of 'going out for the day' living in a place like this?*

I was expecting her to say, 'I've just spent most of the afternoon locked in a cell and I've been screaming the house down. How have you been?'

I saw the Arabic man staring at me. I could sense him undressing me with his intense eyes or seeing more of me than I wanted him to.

I could feel, see and hear everything in the dining area being played in slow motion. I could hear slurping and munching. The smell of the vegetables was overpowering. I heard chairs scraping, noses being blown. I could see particles in the air from the light that was shining through the window. They looked like a cloud of insects that weren't moving. It was as if they had just landed and would be stopping for eternity.

I saw the Arabic man smile at me and I saw his white teeth glistening against his dark skin. His lips were a purple colour and he poked his tongue out and made it curl at the end.

What is wrong with him? God only knows and really I don't want to find out! How can I get better – if there is anything wrong with me – enclosed in a house with lunatics surrounding me? It occurred to me that it wasn't just the patients who were terminally insane but the medical staff too.

I wanted to go to bed early and the nurse said that seeing it was my first night they would allow it. I was told I had to take my medication first. An element of fascism had crept into their lives – I was sure of it. I knew I could not refuse the medication, as I was an inpatient. It didn't make sense that I was in hospital having to ask them for help and then refusing their hospitality. I was trying very hard to figure it all out and as I found this difficult, I thought it best to acquiesce to their judgement. The memory of Glenda and the cell didn't help matters either. I wondered what she did to offend their thinking. That first night I took six tablets. Even when I asked the nurse about the type of chemical cocktail I was about to digest, she responded, 'You'll have to ask your doctor.' They were very skilled in evasive tactics. I hoped, if I was compliant, I would soon be leaving the premises.

I went upstairs to my bedroom, passing the cell-like room again. I looked through my suitcase and noticed my mother had given me a hardback diary. I placed it beside my bed on the chest of drawers.

Suddenly I saw the dark-haired nurse at my door.

'What's that there?' She was looking at my notebook.

I quickly picked it up and held it to my chest. 'Nothing – I don't want you to read it.' Although there was nothing in there to read, I just didn't like the invasion of my privacy. I was paranoid, but then I thought I had a right to be.

She didn't like my response and I saw her eyes grow larger and they were glaring at me. 'All right, have it your way. The men's quarters are down the other end and you are never to go there, understand?' She waited for me to acknowledge her statement and then left the room.

I wondered if she thought me incapable of logical thought or that I didn't understand the English language. I wondered why she was so angry. Was it because I didn't share my thoughts, let her read my diary?

The strong medication was having an effect and as I drifted off to sleep, I tried to visualise a serene image but I couldn't imagine anything. I didn't have time to; the sleeping tablet had worked. I had a restless night, dreaming of locked rooms with small square windows. I saw people or creatures that were half-human and half-animal – dark shadows with glistening white teeth and tongues that could curl around their bodies. I was only fleeting aware of the nightmare when I woke and I tried to block the imagery from my mind.

The next morning when I opened my eyes I saw a nurse standing at the door observing me – then she quickly walked away.

It's a bit like a game: first you see me, then you don't. I wondered how long she had been standing there.

I felt very tired and I went to the wardrobe to put on my new dressing gown and slippers. I opened the door and lo and behold they were not there. *Mum did buy me new clothes, didn't she?*

I dressed into my T-shirt and jeans and went to the shower room to wash my face. I wanted to look clean and respectable. Although I wasn't trying to impress anyone, I thought my chances of leaving were better if I did appear sane. I went back to my bedroom and put on my sandals – it was spring but the hospital had air conditioning so I would be comfortable in that respect. I was still wondering what had happened to my white dressing gown when I went down for breakfast.

I followed the others, selecting a box of cereal, and poured myself a glass of orange juice. I saw the nurse standing at a table ready to administer the medication. She looked like a minister standing at a pew overlooking the congregation. I wondered what her sermon would be.

It wasn't long before I was called and had to swallow various coloured pills.

The nurse had small eyes and small round glasses to match. She reminded me of a crustacean of some sort – an animal that lived in a mollusc or shell with little beady eyes peering out.

'These tablets are supposed to make me feel better, are they?' I said.

'Yes, they should,' the crab-like nurse said.

'Well, how do you know? I mean, what happens?' I thought it was a reasonable question.

'I think you better talk to your doctor about it.'

'My doctor? Who is my doctor anyway?' I had not seen Doctor Grimshaw, or any doctor for that matter.

'Don't you know?' she replied.

Well, obviously not, otherwise I wouldn't be asking the question.

'I don't know who my doctor is and I haven't seen a doctor yet.' I pronounced the words very clearly and made the statement as if I was talking in slow motion.

'Perhaps you just need to settle down. I'll find out who your doctor is and talk to you later, okay?'

Great. She doesn't even know who my doctor is. It's not as if there are two hundred patients in this ward.

I looked about me and I counted twelve 'inmates'. *More evasive tactics.*

'Can I go out? I mean, leave the premises? Go for a walk, that sort of thing?'

Nurse mollusc stared at me as if I had just said something unspeakable. I sounded like I was on some sort of holiday tour and just letting her know I was off and would be back shortly. It felt like surreal hotel accommodation.

'I wouldn't do that, if I was you,' she said.

Okay, why not?

'You're having some tests done today, you have to stay here,' she continued.

Oh, she knows that much but doesn't know who my doctor is.

I realised that I had little choice. I remembered the doctor mentioning detainment. It had not occurred to me that I would be under continual observation and supervision – that I was not allowed even to go out and get some fresh air.

'You mean I have to stay here all the time?' I said.

'You can only leave if accompanied by a nurse,' she said. Nurse mollusc was turning into a very frightening animal.

I gasped. *What have I done to deserve this?*

I sat at the dining table after breakfast wondering what next to do. I think I drank at least fifteen cups of coffee that morning just to keep my eyelids open and my brain working. I watched people – patients talking and some people who were visiting their nearest and dearest. It was fairly quiet, only now and then an argument would erupt and it was usually between the family members and the patient. I could see from my vantage point that it was not the patients' problem but rather the relatives' inability to cope with having to visit someone in a mental hospital. By my understanding, it seemed that the relatives needed hospitalisation more than the patient. It was like watching a very depressing episode of *Days of Our Lives* – except I was in it.

A young bright-eyed perky nurse with a black bob hairstyle and a hooked nose came hurrying up to me. 'It's time for your tests,' she said.

I looked at her and wondered if she had an attitude problem too.

'Yes, you have to come into the interviewing room.'

I didn't have long to wait to find out just what sort of test I was up against. The room was small with a desk and two chairs. I had a feeling of déjà vu. I waited there thinking I would be seeing Doctor Grimshaw again, but I was surprised to see another man enter.

'Hello, I'm Doctor Lish.' He looked older than Doctor Grimshaw and his hair was receding. He wore glasses, black, thick-rimmed spectacles that were far too large for his face. He reminded me of some nutty professor.

'We're just going to do a few tests today, just reporting the day, date, time and place, that sort of thing,' he said.

Report?

His manner was very impersonal. He was robotic as if he was testing the amount of bacterial growth in a test tube. 'I am going to say the name of a fictitious person, where he lives, his street address and his occupation and at the end of this interview, I want you to repeat it back to me, okay?'

I acknowledged the fact that this was a memory test. I nodded.

'Mr James Ogden. He lives at Number 2 Mirrorbank Drive, New Hampstead, and he's an engineer. Okay?'

I nodded. I repeated the facts again in my mind. I was quite good at this sort of thing – it had helped me in school when passing exams.

'Now I want you to take seven from one hundred in descending order – like one hundred, ninety-three, and so on, until you get to zero.

Right, what's the best way of doing this? I saw him look at his watch. *He's counting how long it will take me!*

I thought the easiest way was to take ten from a hundred and then add three. So I started ninety-three, eight-six, seventy-nine, seventy-two, sixty-five, fifty-eight, fifty-one, forty-four, thirty-seven, thirty, twenty-three, sixteen, nine and two. *Was that right?*

I watched him writing. *Was I too slow or had I made mistakes – was he going to tell me?*

'Now I want you to say the months of the year backwards starting with December.'

I thought that was fairly easy. 'November' and I stated the obvious – the other months in sequence.

Then he placed a watch down on the desk in front of me. 'I want you to name the parts and components,' he said, pointing to the face of the watch.

'Watch face or dial?' I said. I felt like I was in some weird game show.

He pointed to the side of the watch.

'Winder.'

'What is that hand that ticks by,' he said.

'Hands, fingers,' I answered.

He pointed to the leather band.

'Strap.'

Then the nutty professor took a pen from his shirt pocket and placed it on the desk. He pointed to it.

'Pen,' I said.

He took off its cap and pointed at that.

'Top.'

Then he pointed at the middle of the pen.

'Barrel.'

Then he pointed at the top of the pen.

'Nib.'

Then he showed me his shoe and pointed to the bottom of it.

'Sole,' I said. At this point I didn't know whether to laugh or to be really afraid. This was all very sinister.

'Now we are going to do some tests with money and arithmetic – name the coins.'

He placed on the table a dollar coin, a twenty-cent piece and a ten-cent piece. I thought it was fairly simple. Then he asked me to add together some sums, which was fairly easy too. Then he gave me some easy division and multiplication sums. I'm pretty sure I answered them all correctly.

'Now for some general knowledge,' he said.

I felt like singing out 'It's the jeopardy special' but this was not a game.

'Who is the prime minister – the preceding prime minister – the premier of this state?'

I answered all the questions correctly – I was quite impressed with my own capabilities by this time.

'What are the capital cities of these countries? France?'

'Paris,' I said.

'Italy?'

'Rome.'

'Japan?'

'Tokyo,' I said.

'Germany?'

'Bonn.' *No it isn't – it's Berlin. Do I get a second chance?*

'Spain.'

'Not sure.'

'Australia.'

'Canberra.' That one was easy.

'Date of last world war?'

'1941.'

'End of war?'

'1945.'

'Name the six largest cities in Australia.'

That was easy too.

'How many cards in a pack of cards?'

'Fifty-two.'

'How many of each sort?'

'Thirteen.'

'Now for some abstract thinking tests,' he said. 'Do you know what a proverb is?'

'Yes, a wise saying,' I replied.

'What does this proverb mean – a rolling stone gathers no moss?'

I had always hated this proverb – it never made sense to me. I was starting to panic. *How can he understand my problem by these measurements? A rolling stone gathers no moss? It was trick question, I was sure of it. What happens if I don't give the appropriate answer? I probably won't win the prize?*

'A person who sits and waits or…? No, it's someone who moves all the time and doesn't get dirty.' *Oh God, I've messed that one up.*

'It's an ill wind that blows nobody any good?'

'If it's sick it doesn't do much for other people,' I said.

'What is the difference between a wall and a fence?'

'One is more solid and the other one is smaller.'

'Ice and glass?'

'Glass you can look through, ice you can't.'

'A child and a dwarf?'

'A dwarf is older but not necessarily but is the same size as a child but then a child can grow taller.'

'What is the name of the man and his address and occupation that I told you earlier?'

'Yes, okay – his name is James Ogden. He lives at Number 2 Mirrorbank Drive, New Hampstead, and he's an engineer.'

'Okay, that will be all for today. You can go back to the ward now.'

'Thank you,' I said and wondered why I was appreciative. I stared at him for a moment, and then got up walked out of the room and back to the day unit. *For the life of me, I have no idea what that was all about.*

I did not want to socialise so I probably did look strange sitting at the dining table for hours on end just staring into space. My isolative behaviour was due to my resistance to their therapy, which to my belief was non-existent except for the medication, and I felt I had little control over that area.

I didn't understand the nurses' hostility. Perhaps it was due to my not liking their methods and they had picked up on my aggression. Their note-taking replaced conversation. The term 'observation' is an apt description. The nurses took different shifts and during my stay I saw at least fifteen different ones. There were different schedules – the morning shift, afternoon shift and the night-time shift. I thought the night-time shift would be the easiest of the three. On occasion when I couldn't sleep and was allowed to get a Milo from downstairs, I would see them in the lounge watching the television. Mind you, I didn't see the other nurses doing a lot of work either, not in the form of actually helping anyone. When I did summon the courage to talk openly to a nurse, I had hoped to have a sympathetic or understanding response.

'I'll be with you in a minute,' the nurse said.

I waited in the dining area, my usual haunt, drinking probably my thirtieth cup of coffee. It was the afternoon and I was hoping my mother would be visiting again today.

The nurse with the black bob hairstyle came back and she sat down next to me. 'Well, Gardenia, how are you?'

'I don't think I'm crazy. I'm just depressed because of the termination.' I thought I'd get straight to the point.

'Do you want to talk about it?' she said.

I looked at her, wondering if that was all she was going to say. 'I don't think I need the medication.' I was sure I was starting to feel the effects of the drugs. I was feeling very tired. I had a dry mouth, no saliva at all. I guess that was why I was drinking copious amounts of coffee. I also couldn't remember when I had last visited the toilet. I wondered if the effects of the medication also made me constipated.

'Are you upset by being here? Not liking the reality of being unwell?'

'I'm not sure – I don't understand what's wrong with me.'

'Don't you? Perhaps you should explain your feelings.'

'I feel confused.

'Are your thoughts bothering you?'

'My thoughts – what do you mean by that? I'm not having any hallucinations, seeing things or hearing voices. Well, I can hear your voice.' I tried to make a joke.

She didn't smile.

'I'm just saying to myself over and over that I'll be all right.'

'I think you're trying to intellectualise your situation and I don't think it's helping you,' she said.

I was frustrated and distressed by her persistent generalisations. She was not giving me any concrete answers. If she could see I was distressed, why didn't she relate some of her knowledge, ideas or reasons for my current fears? Wasn't she trained for that? I was sure my anxieties were not just the result of being in a mental hospital. There was something more to it, surely. Had she given me some reassurance, to reinforce I was okay, perhaps my life would have been different. Instead, the nurses were doing exactly the opposite, reinforcing my self-doubt, my inadequate coping skills. They were in fact saying I was mentally ill. I was continually getting the impression that they were trying to understand me but I was not giving them the right answers. This in itself was confusing and only increased my sense of powerlessness and my tendency to withdraw from any social interaction.

After this conversation, I decided to try and do something. I played a game of eight ball – albeit on my own, but it was a start. I had just placed the balls in the triangle when I suddenly felt my head move to the side. It was a strange feeling having my head at right angles to my body. I tried to move it back but I couldn't. I stood there not knowing what to do. Should I call for help? I had no idea of what was happening. Quickly a nurse ran up to me and led me to a treatment room. At least they were competent with their observation skills. A doctor hurried in to see me, and after a few moments when he had injected some chemical into my system, the paralysis went away. I heard the doctor say the word 'cogentin'. That was the only answer I was given in relation to the event. At the time, I thought that it was part of my illness, that I was really losing my marbles and this was an example of the process. I didn't know at the time that it was a reaction to the medication. They could have said that at least.

My mother came and visited me soon afterwards. I was looking forward to her visit but when I saw her, I started crying. Her presence reminded me of home and being away from this environment. The fact that I was locked up in here was increasing my depression.

'What's wrong, Gardenia?'

I probably didn't look very well. I had seen the dark circles under my eyes and I didn't think I was looking any better for being in hospital.

'Have you been eating?' she said.

I nodded. I had only been eating the dessert. 'I think someone stole my dressing gown,' I said.

'Yes, they told me when I came in, but they've found your clothes and they're back in your room. Have you settled in and are they helping you?'

I nodded. I felt like I was on my own and that I had to pretend I was getting better – it was the only way of escaping this place.

'I think there's a man here, a Middle Eastern chap who has sexual problems,' I said. I didn't like telling tales, but then I didn't like him showing me his genitals either.

'What sexual problems, Gardenia?'

'He likes flashing,' I said.

'Oh, God.'

'I'm sorry, Mum.' There wasn't much more I could say. I hated making her distressed.

I wanted to tell her about the nutty professor and how I had to tell him he had a sole at the bottom of his shoe, but I was too tired to form the words. After some time, my mother left saying she would be back the next day. We hadn't talked that much – she just sat with me, as I stared into nothingness. *I'm just making life difficult for her. I wonder if she'll be back to visit me again.*

The next morning I was so tired I couldn't even move. The nurses helped me get up by pushing me out of bed and holding me either side and walking me to the shower cubicle. It was like torture as I leaned on the wall unaware of the water falling on my body. My inability to wake up made me feel I was in some sort of trance. I had never felt so exhausted in my life.

This extreme fatigue gradually lifted and I tried to do something constructive. I went to the craft room and painted a ceramic figurine. The two patients who were also contemplating the joy of mass-produced clay figures said that there was to be a game of bingo that afternoon – so I was really looking forward to that.

The hospital was like a large operating room – a clinical observation post. Surgery was being performed everyday in the ward – notes taken, medication given. The only thing to be aware of was the patients' state of mind – whether the interaction of the medication was working or if it needed to be changed or increased. To define a person's state of mind was a matter of conjecture. It was the medical staff's informed opinion that made the decision of a person's sanity. Obviously the patients in this hospital were medically unfit to resume an independent life.

The day room had comfortable seats and sofas but they were taken up continually by the other patients. I was very tired and the only seating available consisted of the hard-edged dining room chairs. Sometimes I sat on the grey carpeted floor in the corner of the room near the window. I didn't want to get into an argument – having to fight for my right to sit in a cushioned chair. Although I was very tired, my anxiety was spiralling. I could literally feel my body trembling. My hands were shaking – a visible tremor and this made it difficult for me to pick up the coffee mug without spilling it.

That night I wrote in my diary.

> It is not surprising that my medication has tripled, given my deterioration. Although I do not know what the pills are for, or why they are giving them to me. I am too afraid now to ask and no one thinks to tell me. I can see the nurses watching me and I don't dare talk to any of the patients – I'm scared what they will write down about me. I will keep on saying I'm all right to myself over and over and I'm sure I will get better. I only have to wait another four days and I will be home.

My mother visited me again the next day. She said that she had been talking to the medical staff and had asked to see a private psychiatrist. I think my mother disliked the treatment I was receiving. She said they had agreed to this, but I had my doubts. I finally did have a consultation with the private psychiatrist. I thought I would be visiting the specialist in his private rooms, but he came to the hospital. I was sure that he was a part of Felixstowe Hospital and as such I doubted whether his opinion would be different. I did try to make him understand that I was okay and that I didn't need help. It was as if I was making a plea for my freedom. That I had not done anything wrong, that I did not need to sit in front of a jury. Why was I being judged? I made sure I answered all his questions appropriately, in a reasonable and rational manner. I still had no idea what they were writing or what the medication consisted of or whether or not I was going to be discharged.

On the sixth day of my stay, I was starting to feel better, knowing I would be discharged the next day.

'I'm going home tomorrow,' I said to the nurse.

'Are you? It isn't written in the notes.'

My heart sank – this was not going to be easy. 'They said I only needed to stay for a week.'

'Did they? Perhaps your doctor needs to make sure about that.' It wasn't nurse mollusc but they were beginning to look and sound all the same.

'I'm a volunteer patient. You have no reason to keep me here.'

I stayed another two days but I was only allowed to go home under my mother's care. I had to come back in a week's time for a follow-up consultation. I had to sign an 'own risk consent' form. My vision had deteriorated and I suspected it was because of the medication. Reading was difficult, but I could just make out the words:

This certifies that I the undersigned leave the hospital against the advice of the medical officer in charge of my case and I hereby agree not to hold the hospital authorities responsible for any harm or injury that may result from my action.

I signed the document.

My mother and I had to go to the hospital pharmacy to collect my medication. I was taking fluphenazine, a major tranquilliser or antipsychotic, as well as orphenadrine, a treatment used in Parkinson's disease, also useful as a muscle relaxant (this was used to counteract the effects of the fluphenazine – tremors and paralysis); lorazepam, an antianxiety drug; temazepam, a sleeping pill. Senokot was added to the mix for my severe constipation.

I had to keep alert enough to make sure I understood the types of medication I was being told to digest. It was the only way of understanding my illness or what they thought I was suffering from. It was also very important to understand their ideas and hence treatment. I realised that the hospital was not a place where miraculous cures were made. Neither was it a place where recovery was possible. It was a morbid, strange hell and I was very glad to leave it. It was a cold place that tried to make you believe it was warm. Its veneer was shiny but underneath, the wood was rotten. The smiles were sweet but the words were foul.

I knew they thought I was mentally unfit. I tried to clasp on to my own strength – to believe in my own sanity. I had cooperated with their system while still trying to keep my self belief and self worth. I had spent my twenty-first birthday in hospital – my mother was my only visitor.

*

Felixstowe Hospital
Outpatient records
Doctor G. Grimshaw

Gardenia Baxter
The patient is not experiencing acute psychotic
symptoms. Her reactive response is adequate and she is
lucid and cooperative. She is reactive to situations
and conversation - mixing in well, playing games and
communicating appropriately on a superficial level.
No evidence of thought disorder although she has a
depressive mood and is tearful, sad. 'She states she
is depressed about being in hospital and wants to
start work and do things'.
No suicidal ideation.
Her affect continues to be blunt and at particular
times becomes quite angry. Also makes inappropriate
comments. Her withdrawn behaviour 'inability to talk'
may be due to thought blocking 'hearing voices or
seeing things'.

Has difficulty with abstract thought - takes a long
way around to get to the point and tends to talk
on a tangent. Her confusion is still apparent with
disorganised associations - possibly displaying a
certain type of schizophrenic disorder.
Mrs Baxter requested referral to see private
psychiatrist. Dr Long agreed with treatment plan and
referred patient back to duty doctor. Mrs Baxter's
continual interference and her constant need for
confirmation that her daughter is all right is making
treatment of Gardenia difficult. She may need to learn
to direct her concerns to other matters with mutual
benefit for her and patient. Mrs Baxter needs education
of Gardenia's disorder as Gardenia lacks subjective
thought.
To be discharged under care of mother and notified Mrs
Baxter of the possibility of respite if warranted.
To return in a week's time to see duty doctor as an
outpatient.
Continuing Fluphenazine 5 mg. morning and night.
Lorazepam prn.
Temazepam 10-20 mg at night. Orphenadrine 50 mg
morning and night.

Signed
Dr G. Grimshaw

7

I was glad to be home, yet the admission had made an impact on me. The self-doubt and worry had not ceased. Living at home in a somewhat normalised or rational environment made me hopeful that things could get better, although I questioned the aspect of what 'normality' actually meant. During the next month, I tried not think of myself as having a mental illness, which was not easy

I decided to continue practising my art, painting and drawing. The possibility of generating an income inspired me, even if the reality of it happening was tenuous. In the local paper I saw an advert relating to an exhibition project initiated by the government for those who were unemployed. I decided to participate.

In a different setting with other like-minded artists, I was able to accomplish more than I first thought possible, even selling one painting at the final exhibition. The painting depicted a Queensland forest. I used acrylics, a smooth buttery-type mixture that I liked. Mixtures of greens and purples dominated the scene with the tall trees. Their long straight trunks were a creamy purple colour rising into the sky. A canopy of dark green leaves weaved around the tree trunks. The colours merged in an impressionistic way with the opening space of the background sky. The light touched the delicate foreground bushes with orange and pink highlights. I enjoyed creating this serenity. I could be a part of another world and it made a difference, if only for a short while. The woman who bought the painting said it reminded her of home. She came from Canada.

I still suffered with acute anxiety and panic attacks, struggling to make sense of my thoughts and feelings but I needed to prove my capacity to function as a 'normal' human being. I was at first sceptical that I would be able to cope, meeting new people, catching buses. I did feel uncomfortable at first but there were three other girls participating, all ex-graduates of an art school. I soon understood we had common interests.

My nervousness and social anxiety lessened as the young women did not question my history or evaluate me as anything but a person interested in art. The government gave us money for materials, paints, canvases and so on. One day we made an expedition to the Dandenong Forest. I travelled in a bright red Volkswagen with the three other girls. Georgina owned the car and she was adamant about having direct access with nature, to be inspired, she said. I took photos of the landscape, taking in the subtle colours, the vibrancy of the green ferns. I watched the sulphur-crested cockatoos and rosella parrots squawking at tourists who loved to continually feed their ravenous appetites. I used these images later for my paintings. During this time, I forgot about Felixstowe and my own problems. I was lost in another sphere, making sense of an outside world that was beautiful.

My fears would return each time I walked through the Felixstowe gates, knowing I would be under constant evaluation with the doctors' pressing questions. I feared the possibility of going mad and being confined in the hospital. I felt like a jellyfish that had been caught, lying on parched sand barely able to breathe. I wanted someone to pick me up and put me in the ocean, tell me I was okay. I didn't want to be a fish out of water.

I continued to see Doctor Grimshaw as an outpatient once a week. I was still taking the medication, but was worried by the implications – what was wrong with me, so to speak. Doctor Grimshaw was still talking in riddles. I was not getting anywhere in obtaining answers, but he seemed to be very interested in my thinking. I tried hard to go back to a former way of life or time. I even went to personal growth courses to help my social anxieties. I tried to forget the hospital, the doctors and the diagnosis of mental illness.

My attempts to try and ignore the recent past, the termination and my generalised fears meant I was denying important feelings and emotions. In my mind I was creating a new identity – playing the role of another person. My reasons for trying to formulate another personality were due to the fact that I had lost something intrinsically important. I knew who I was, my name and where I lived. I knew the reality of my surroundings, but when it came to understanding the bricks and mortar of my personality, well, that was irretrievable. This was not just a case of questioning my place in society or what I wanted from life – this was a major debilitating and profound problem. The core or essence of my mind, soul, and character had disappeared. I lived in a fog, a cloudy unreal universe. I was blind, trying to hold onto something solid. It was like being submerged under water and learning to swim in quicksand.

It was difficult to describe this terror – this lost world I inhabited. I could not explain my pain – it was something that could not even be known. It was a void, an eternity of nothing, a blank space, and I lived in it.

The conversations with Doctor Grimshaw only intensified my dilemma. My attempts to pretend I was okay reinforced my belief that I was not. My inability to remember or concentrate meant I stumbled with my words and on occasion found it difficult to even conceptualise a thought. I lived in the present moment and as such my comprehension was limited.

I wanted to believe that it was the medication that was creating my problem and I think it did exacerbate my difficulties. It's difficult to speculate whether the increased dosages of medication caused my symptoms, or if in fact my aberration was the reason. It is impossible to know what my life would have been like without the treatment.

My physical body was feeling the effects of the medication, although in my own confusion I understood it as being a part of my illness. Although my emotional life was in turmoil, I still had enough intelligence to realise my circumstances – a life in ruins. I was not interested in living a life of pain. Who would be?

The tremors in my hands and arms continued, as did my falling over, tripping on the rough pavement as I walked to the local shops with my mother. My muscular impairment, falling flat on my face time and time again, made me cry and this emotional response was so intense that I believed I was going insane. It was frightening especially when walking down the stairs – I had to be careful not to fall.

My panic attacks were so overwhelming that often I could not even walk a hundred metres and would turn back home, relieved to have the protection and security of something I knew.

I didn't know the cause of such attacks, only that I felt threatened. People in general scared me and I felt a sense of disassociation as if I was somewhere else, like an out of body experience. My breathing would increase as I took in short bursts of oxygen. My stomach would churn and my heart would beat rapidly as if I had just played a high-energy sport. I literally thought I was going to die. This unusual reaction contradicted my reasons for having a happy social experience. Going to the cinema with my mother was an event that bordered on torture.

When I started to experience epilepsy, I again thought it was due to my illness. My extreme feelings of despair had not reasoned it could be anything else. The fit usually took on the appearance of falling unconscious, although I was aware of my arms frantically shaking. One day, when I was on a ladder, lifting boxes from the top of a wardrobe, I had another unexpected fit. I fell, hitting my head rather badly, causing lacerations and loss of blood. The paramedics who had previously seen my psychiatric history had reasoned that it was due to hyperventilation and anxiety. The doctors at Felixstowe had noted these attacks, but were hesitant to diagnose me with any concrete disorder – although they did refer me to a neurologist to understand the cause.

I saw the specialist at Felixstowe Hospital. I returned to the same ward, the place where I had first been hospitalised. I walked through the sliding automatic doors once more into the day ward, to wait again in the reception area for my appointment.

The neurologist was a tall man with dark hair. He was more likeable than the other doctors I had seen – Doctor Grimshaw and the nutty professor. Perhaps it was because my opinion of him was different or my perception that possibly he could have some answers.

'I'm Doctor Spook. Can you tell me what happened? I see here you had a fall.'

'I was out the back and climbing on a ladder so I could get some boxes from on top of a wardrobe and I fell, just like that. I think I must have blacked out.'

'What did it feel like when you fell?' he said.

'Like a loss of movement,' I said.

'What happened?'

'I just went blank and fell unconscious but I did see my arms moving wildly around.'

I want you to walk down the passageway and back again,' he said. I knew he was studying me and I felt my body, the way I walked, was all wrong. I was robotic in movement. I felt like a deranged zombie or Doctor Frankenstein's monster because I was sure my arms were supposed to swing. My arms were stuck to my sides. Perhaps I had to walk in a hurry for my arms to move?

Like the other doctors, he didn't give me any answers. He didn't even try to give me reassurance. He just liked to ask questions and that was it. I had no idea at that time that the medication I was on lowered the threshold for epileptic fits. He asked me a few questions, similar to the other tests I had undergone. The arithmetic of taking seven from one hundred again.

'What time is it?' He pointed to the clock on the wall.

'Two-thirty,' I said. Of course I knew that. 'I have a continuous muscular spasm,' I said.

'Where?'

'In my arm.' I saw him look at my now static arm. 'I also tremble and have restlessness in my arms and legs and I feel so anxious at times I feel like climbing the walls.' I watched him writing his notes.

'I have irregular periods too – only one in the last six months. I also have severe constipation. I have to go to accident and emergency once a week to have an enema. Those chemist alternatives, the syrup and the grains and the horrible prunes – they don't work.'

'It must be difficult,' he said.

115

I knew he wouldn't be interested in such problems but it needed to be said and I hoped that if he wrote it down, possibly something could be done. I didn't tell him how humiliating it was having young inexperienced nurses laugh at me as they squirted detergent up my nether regions.

I had looked for alternatives, wondering if herbal medicines would relieve my condition. I spent hours in chemist shops and in the library trying to evaluate the benefits of vitamin B or the effects of evening primrose oil. I had now assumed I was going through some midlife crisis, except I was experiencing it early. Also I suspected that I was either going through some extreme premenstrual tension, or menopause had set in.

The well intentioned drug companies were making a packet out of me. Every concoction, liver diets, cleansing systems, nerve tonics were part of my regime. Menopause relief tablets were also on my ever-increasing list of medications. I physically felt myself rattling. The benefits? There weren't any.

My vision had also deteriorated, so I had to wear prescription glasses. I looked like a person wearing binoculars – the lenses were so thick you could have mistaken them for bottles.

My frequent angry outbursts directed at my mother gave me some release and God knows I apologised for them, time and again. She understood, I don't know how, but she did.

I often tried to talk to my mother about my condition. 'I'm not going to do their bloody rehabilitation,' I said.

'That's okay, Gardenia, you don't have to.'

'Yes, but I do, don't you see? They've pushed me into a corner.'

'I don't think so. They're just trying to help.'

'I can't concentrate – I feel stuck in the house not getting anywhere. How can I expect to go back to uni or live a life with that label – psychotic? Do they want me to be that? Should I tell them they're right? Shall I do something to make them give me a terminal chemical lobotomy, because that's what it is, isn't it? I can't read because I can't see. I can't even watch television because I'm so agitated. I've lost my life, my happiness. Does that make sense to you?'

My mother in her wisdom just listened.

'They just want to probe, figure out what's going on in my mind. They just won't listen, will they? They just want to prove their theories. Am I intellectualising my condition or are they the ones doing that? I'm a scientific experiment and they're saying it's for the benefit of the patient. I mean, what are they writing about me? I can't even physically function and they think I'm paranoid.'

Usually after a confrontation such as this I would go to my bedroom, slam the door and say I was going to kill myself or some other dramatic inappropriate emotional response. I usually ended up saying sorry to my mother – that I was no good, that I was sick. She would then tell me that I wasn't sick, that I just needed rest and that everything would be all right. I wanted to give her my glasses to see – perhaps they would have made a difference.

When I calmed down, I would try and explain my position logically to her. 'Every two weeks they have different ideas, and they change my medication and dosages frequently. I don't think it's good to be changing the drugs all the time, especially in connection to the mind, do you? For example, what happens if you mix too many alcoholic drinks?'

'I don't know, Gardenia.'

'You'd throw up, wouldn't you?'

'I really want to help but I just don't know what to do.' I watched my mother mixing the flour and milk – she was making lemonade scones.

'I answer all the questions correctly, don't I? How can I be psychotic or insane or whatever and still go to my course or paint or get on the bus? How can I be both things at once?'

'But they don't think you're like that, Gardenia,' said my mother.

'What? You must be joking.'

'You know they're student doctors,' said my mother.

'What? They're not even trained psychiatrists?'

'Well, technically no, but they are in their last year of studies to become a psychiatrist,' my mother continued.

'So they don't have any experience at all?' I said, completely horrified but not really surprised.

'No, but students can pick up on things that learned doctors might miss,' she said.

'I think they're missing a brain and that's an understatement.'

I did understand my mother's passivity, because her hands were tied. Who could she go to for support? She didn't want to increase my frustration, but to alleviate it. I needed her help and she was doing the best she could.

I hoped Doctor Grimshaw would tell me I only had some anxiety and depression and prescribe appropriate antidepressants. He would then encourage me to use some psychological self-help tools, to be on my way. But that was not to be the case.

A week had gone by quickly and I waited again in the reception area at Felixstowe for my appointment with the duty doctor. I looked at Doctor Grimshaw and noticed his nose was far too long for his face but his eyes suggested that he was healthy – they were bright and clear. At once I felt displeasure with his manner and attitude. He had not changed and was continuing to treat me with a certain kind of contempt, as if I was a basket case and should be treated as such.

'Hello, and your thoughts today, how are they?'

Did he say be brave? He spoke so quickly, I only had time to understand the word 'they'.

'So how have you been? How are your thoughts today?' He spoke slower this time – perhaps he could see by my furrowed brow that I had trouble in understanding him?

Do you want a long answer or a short one? I thought.

'I'm so tired in the mornings that I don't know whether I should have a shower first or eat my breakfast before a shower or get dressed before I have breakfast.' *I should get dressed after a shower, that's the right order, isn't it?*

He was already scribbling down something.

Okay, I'm dyslectic, so what?

'The idea of doing anything makes it difficult for me to think,' I said. *No, I should have said I find it difficult to think, so I can't do anything.*

'What are you frightened of, Gardenia?'

You – but was he referring to something specific? 'I don't know – I suppose it's just that I am. Really, I don't know.' I had forgotten the question.

'Have you had thoughts of suicide?' he asked. I saw his scalp – his hair was thinning.

'No, not recently.'

'So you have had those thoughts then?'

I knew he was going to say that. I didn't answer and I watched him as he wrote more notes regarding my mental state.

'What are you thinking of now?'

I didn't say anything again because I was confused by the first question about being frightened of something but I didn't know what.

I remembered my last effort – telling him I was tired and couldn't get up in the mornings. 'I find it hard to get out of bed,' I said.

'Why is that?'

'Because I'm tired,' I said. I knew it was a simple response, so I tried to sound more enthusiastic. 'I am getting better although I've been trying very hard to cope with daily activities, just household duties – cleaning, cooking and helping my mother.'

'Have you given any thought to the rehabilitation scheme we've outlined for you, to go back to the work force?'

I wondered if he had read the labels on these tablets. The words that spell out you can't operate any machinery or drive a vehicle. I felt like I couldn't do anything really. *I mean, what happens if I have an unexpected fit crossing the road?* I really did think they were morons.

'I don't think I'm ready at this time – I still have social anxieties,' I said.

'Would you like to live in a halfway house or community house?'

Would you?

'I've had it!' I shouted at him. 'I do not want to do your programme, okay?' I got up and stormed out. I stood by the front entrance near the sliding automatic door and watched it open and then close and then open again.

I recognised my mistake. *This is not a good thing to do, to show them I'm angry.*

I went back to the interviewing room.

'I'm glad you came back, Gardenia. Have you been angry like this with your mother too?'

I nodded. I knew I had been making my mother's life difficult.

'Do you think it might be a good idea to come into hospital?'

'No, I'll be all right.' I could feel tears welling up in my eyes. I didn't want him to see me crying.

'Have you been going out or just staying around the house?'

'I've been going to a community centre and learning to paint. I'm trying to fathom watercolour at the moment.'

I could see his eyes glaze over.

'I don't think I'm very good – trying to mix the colours so they don't get too dark like a blobby mess. I have a friend who I occasionally go out with. We went to a barbecue and I had a couple of glasses of wine. I enjoyed it.'

'How many glasses of wine did you have?'

'Six, I think, but it could have been five or seven – I can't remember.'

'You had that much wine?' He looked at me as if my very presence made him want to vomit some disgusting muck from his chest.

'Yes.'

'Don't you realise what that could do to you?'

I felt like saying the same back to him – that the amount of pills I was taking was making me very sick. I controlled my tongue – I was learning to stay focused and not to say anything that would unduly cause them to lock me up.

'I am trying to cope, you know, making inroads really, with my silk painting and pottery. I've been to my lessons and I've been going to those groups – you know, for the unemployed. I get very tired and can't concentrate for long.' I watched his nose twitch and wondered if he had a broomstick hidden somewhere. *They have male witches, don't they?*

'I don't feel up to doing a lot but I do try. I really don't think I need to take the fluphenazine any more. I don't think it's helping me – it makes me very tired.' *God, that took a lot of effort and courage!*

'I see.'

'Also I think the tranquilliser makes me depressed and I can't think. I'd like to read a book, but I'm just too tired.' I wondered if he'd got the point yet.

'I can see by your glasses that you're having problems with your vision,' he said.

I wonder if that's a trick question.

'Yes.' *He has impeccable insight.*

'I feel like people are laughing at me,' I said.

'Really?'

'Yes, it's not nice going to the hospital every week to have an enema and have nurses laughing behind my back. Actually, they don't care if I hear them. People think I'm a nutcase – I just know it.'

'How do you know that?'

I could see he wanted to finish this session – he was looking at his watch. I couldn't answer that question – it was a bit like do you know how your thoughts happen? *If I could answer that, I suppose I'd know the meaning of life.*

'Do you think I like putting suppositories up my bottom every day? To continually put those insertion things in my anus and using haemorrhoid cream and my mother just saying you need to relax? Also I have a dry mouth, does that have something to do with it, like no moisture in my body?'

'Perhaps you do need to relax,' he said.

I stared at him, trying to understand how his brain worked or if it did work at all.

'I've had one menstrual period in the last six months.'

'And does that worry you?'

Now I knew he didn't have a brain.

'Perhaps you might be pregnant?'

Wouldn't I be looking fairly large at six months pregnant? I chose not to even answer that question. 'No, I'm not worried about it.' I was sure if he saw me getting more uptight then the pills were going to be increased again.

'Perhaps we better give you a pregnancy test just to make sure?'

I nodded. I couldn't beat his insensible ideas.

'You don't want to be pregnant at the moment, do you?' He laughed.

I realised he had just tried to make a joke and I thought it might be in my best interests to laugh. So I did. He liked my response because it was the first time I saw him smile.

Again I felt persecuted for my termination – that I was promiscuous. I already loathed myself for becoming pregnant in the first place. Did he think I was going to go through all that again?

'I don't know why my arms and hands shake all the time and I even feel my head rattling,' I said.

'Oh yes, I see.'

'Why do I fall and black out?' I said. I watched him shuffle through my file that was now one-quarter-inch thick in size.

'The neurologist has noted that he considers you are not suffering any epilepsy of an organic nature. But we will start you on carbamazepine just to make sure,' he said.

'Oh, that's good,' I said. 'That I don't have epilepsy.' *Carbamazepine – what's that again?*

I was trying to sort through my mind the many medications I had been taking. It had only been a month since my first admission and I had already been on five different types. It was important for me to remember. It was vital, so I could stay on track, to order my mind. To know what the tablets meant and what they did.

It was as if he read my thoughts.

'It can work as a mood stabiliser but it is also useful in epilepsy,' he said.

But I don't have epilepsy or a mood disorder – what does it mean to be stabilised anyway?

'Is a mood stabiliser for manic depression so you don't get too happy or too sad?' I said.

'Yes, something like that.' He looked at his watch again.

I'm sorry if I'm taking up your precious time.

'But I'm never happy.'

'It can work in other ways too,' he said.

I knew he was not going to give me any further explanation.

'Oh, and I see you had a scan for epilepsy. It says you had a scar on your brain.'

Yes, it was another test I was forced into. At least I have a brain, better to have one than not at all.

'So what do you do at home during the day?' he asked.

'I suppose I watch television a lot. I've been watching comedy videos. Mostly American – light-hearted stuff but it's really funny. I think I get a bit obsessed with it but I find it helps. You know, Gene Wilder and young Frankenstein, how he puts the wrong brain in Frankenstein picking up the one that says Abby Normal.'

I don't think he was amused by my attempt at light conversation.

'What else do you do think about?' he asked.

I really didn't know what he expected me to say. I was not aware of my thoughts on a continual basis – they were just automatic.

'I sit outside in the garden and just look at the trees and plants.' Hoping my description of something physical would take him away from the topic of 'thoughts'.

'What do you see in the garden?' he asked.

'Clothes on a rack, moving, turning in the wind,' I said.

He started writing furiously again. I wondered what was so interesting about seeing the washing on the line.

'I think I'm just confused. My memory isn't very good.' It was a logical explanation for my presence in a psychiatrist's interviewing room. I preferred that diagnosis to whatever he was writing, because I knew it wasn't a glowing reference. 'I think I do need to be on medication,' I said. Hoping this would make me appear sane. I feared the consequences. 'Also I think an antidepressant would be a good idea.' *Now I am really sounding enthusiastic.*

'Why is that?' he asked.

'I think it's to do with my abortion. I'm still feeling bad about it.'

'Okay, that might be a good idea. I'll start you on imipramine. Also I think we need to place you on another tranquilliser,' he said. 'I think that you're getting more confused. I'm going to prescribe haloperidol. Also I want you to think about coming back into hospital.'

God, I'd like to throw him out of the window. What's in the garden, Doctor Grimshaw? Are the plants talking to you and how do you feel about that? Can you define it?

I came away feeling I had just been hypnotised. He had proved to me once more that I was insane. How else could I see it? He was going to give me more medication – it was an open and shut case. This had gone too far. I felt I was playing into their hands. It was an ultimatum. This conflict in my mind – the aspect of questioning their authority while also being subjected to it – caused me to continually worry about my future. How could I assert my rights? *Doctor Grimshaw is basically saying that I'm deteriorating. How can I stand up against them?* I could not see any light that would lead me out of this darkness. I succumbed and I was admitted to Felixstowe Psychiatric Hospital.

*

```
Outpatient Records
Doctor Grimshaw

Gardenia Baxter
She is cleanly dressed and cooperative but has dark
rings under her eyes - does not look very well. Also
has dilated pupils.
Her mornings are bad and she doesn't know what to do -
first dress, shower or have breakfast.
Spontaneous slowness of speech but still has loose
associations and bizarre delusions.
Helps mother around home.
Evidence of continued thought disorder, stalked out of
interviewing room - later was tearful.
She refuses to come into hospital but possibly would
```

be interested in half-way house or community house.
She is an uninteresting person and only talks about
art.
Gardenia went to BBQ feels isolated and lonely. Drank
six glasses of wine and she told me this! Advised her
not to do this.
She occupies herself with pottery, silk painting and
goes to unemployed courses. Also has been watching TV.
Mildly psychotic; believes people are laughing at her.
Gardenia expressed her concern for physical symptoms
- arms and hands shaking and her inability to
concentrate. She hears 'ratting in her head'. Also
complains of dry mouth.
But is reassured by neurological examination.
Has not had menstrual period for last 6 months.
Possibly pregnant? Arrange test.
Has spontaneous flow of speech but still has loose
associations. Has good affect - is able to laugh at my
joke but on the whole seems childlike.
Has thought disorder with visual hallucinations -
auditory. Has preoccupation with things she sees on
TV. Had seen clothes moving on a rack in wind.
Correctly understands that she needs her medication.
Has little eye contact but is coherent enough to
express her concerns about her medication.
She continues to feel sad, tired, withdrawn, and
anxious but doesn't know why.
Mood weepy - has diurnal mood variation. Not motivated,
withdrawn. Talks about abortion and her frustration -
anger and rejection.
Obviously needs grief work and to do so without
mother's interference.
Her angry moods have created possible crisis in family
- parental relationship is strained.
She is depressed and thought disordered today - she is
paranoid agitated and angry.
Long conversation produces increased thought disorder.
New symptoms - falling and loss of power in both arms
and headaches. Does she have a history of epileptic
fits?
Has a long way of going about saying something -
doesn't get to the point. Takes time to talk back to

answer questions - perhaps thought blocking due to
hallucinating.
Her communication and thoughts have improved.
Conversation is poor.
Mother reports steady progress.
Impression she remains psychotic.
Continue with medications as same.
Fluphenazine, temazepam, orphenadrine, lorazepam.
To commence haloperidol and imipramine.
Increase fluphenazine.

Outpatient Records
Neurological Examination
Doctor Spook

Gardenia Baxter
Gardenia falls outside - hurts her head and noticed
that her hand trembled. Collapsed loss of movement
- 'went blank'. Also has fallen on several occasions
- seen in accident and emergency they stated,
hyperventilation and anxiety attack.
Also Gardenia is not a particularly good historian and
her insights are poor - is slow to comprehend.
No past history of faints.
A lowered arm swing particularly on the right -
abnormal. Arm weakness must be functional - no
investigations.
Last attack - not of epileptic origin but may have
related to hyperventilation.
Neurological signs of examination unremarkable.
Suggest the addition of carbamazepine.
I would be happy to reassess if necessary.

Signed
Doctor Spook

8

Inpatient records
Doctor Grimshaw

Gardenia Baxter

List of deficits and problems
Previous episode of illness
Ceased own medication
Family - Gardenia's mother is intrusive
Severity of presentation remains psychotic

Lists of assets
Pre morbid function good
Good response to medication
Mother supportive

Admission list
Legal rights and description for detained patients -
need full signature and statement of particulars. Back
of detention paper needs full signature.
Valuables, private medication, potentially harmful
objects - need full signature.
Orientate patient and relatives to ward.
Give guidelines - need full signature.

*

I walked in through the double doors of Felixstowe and was admitted. I had to go through the same sort of paperwork but there were not so many questions this time, because they had already much of the information on hand, personal details, health care card numbers and so on.

I saw the same nurses again – the young tall dark-haired nurse who didn't like me because I didn't show her my diary. The nurse with the black bob haircut who appeared nice but really wasn't. Even the same patients were there – Glenda, Jim and the Arabic man. It had been a month since my first hospital stay and I wondered if they were ever going to be discharged?

I had the same bedroom and only went up there to place my suitcase beside by the bed. I didn't want to stay up there too long and be told off for going against the rules. I wanted my stay to be short. I wondered if it was now okay to be in the bedrooms during the day, but I didn't think they would have changed their rules overnight.

I saw a nurse who was quite different to the rest. She had a vivacious personality and seemed to be happy to be a nurse – she even smiled. I had not seen that before.

'I'm Lucy. How have you been getting on?' she asked.

'Oh, I'm getting better – just to be here makes a big difference,' I lied. 'I won't be here long – just so I can get better and go home.' I didn't know what the nurse expected me to say. *Let's have a martini and play a game of backgammon, hey?*

I was admitted in the morning at the appropriate time between nine-thirty and ten-thirty. I didn't know what to do, so I sat down at the other end of the unit near the long tall windows. I had hoped to be inconspicuous. *I don't have to talk to them – anything I say would be misconstrued. I can't tell the truth. I don't want to get into trouble, telling them I don't trust them. If I do that or say I'm not well, it will imply that I need further hospitalisation.*

I tried to focus my mind on other things and looked out of the window. I watched the lorikeets in the native bottlebrush; as I couldn't hear them, I imagined their squawking. I remembered my own garden at home, sitting out the back, seeing the rosellas in the fig tree. I could see that there was a slight breeze and I noticed the delicate parts of the bottlebrush flowers were moulting and flying into the air. I could see gum trees in the distance, their leaves a mass of shadow against the cobalt blue sky.

I felt like a person who wasn't needed. Like someone in an old persons' home staring out of a window, waiting to die. I could see myself being plied with medication to keep me quiet. To make life easier for them so I wouldn't be a bother. I had never thought in my wildest dreams that I would end up like this. I felt sorry now for all the old people in nursing homes with their frailty and vulnerability, having to be controlled by other people's personalities.

I could see the leaves scattered over the ground, forming mulch. In some places, the red clay soil was cracked, unable to hold any moisture. Water was scarce. Garden lawns were a luxury the community could not afford. I wondered if it was possible to set the hospital grounds on fire. I thought it would be easy to do – drop a lit cigarette, especially in the dry summer heat. I imagined a Hans Heysen painting with cattle walking on a dry path. The brown colours and pale, curled-up bark of the trees. The scene could also be interpreted as an impressionist painting with the constantly changing images, the colour and light moving like small stars. I understood why Van Gogh painted his circling vibrant images.

That day I had to go through another one of those reality tests, or cognitive tests as they are called. I had the same arithmetic test counting backwards from a hundred again by seven. This time I said I was tired, so he allowed me to count backwards by three – which was easier. The test wasn't as extensive as the first.

'What is the difference between ice and glass?'

It was the same question as before but I think I answered it differently.

'Ice is cold and glass cuts,' I said.

'Why should people not throw stones in glasshouses?'

'People in closed situations would hurt each other,' I replied.

'What is the date today?'

'It's the thirtieth of December 1986,' I said.

I found out later that I was one day out when I asked the nurse what day it was. It was the first of January 1987. I hoped they wouldn't hold it against me.

The doctor asked me who the prime minister and premier were, which I still knew, 'although they do change quickly these days,' I said.

That was the end of that round of questioning so I went back to the day room wondering how I was going to cope.

Time went surprisingly quickly and teatime was the next item on the agenda. I think the mealtimes were the most interesting times, involving something practical – although not necessarily pleasant. I was sitting contemplating eating the bread and butter pudding when a nurse who I had never seen before came over with a plate of roast dinner. She put it down beside me.

'I know you want me to eat but I'm not hungry,' I said.

She sat down and I could tell she was going to be persistent. 'But Gardenia, you must eat – it will help.'

I thought she was going to push the spoon in my mouth and treat me like baby. I could spurt it out in her face and say 'Goo.' *No, I shouldn't do that.*

'Just a little bit, Gardenia. I really don't have time to do this, you know – I have work to do, so please eat.'

'God, okay,' I said. Just to have her leave, I would eat the bloody dish of roast beef, peas and carrots that were swimming in the thin gravy. *Talk about coercion.*

I knew then that I was going to die – it was just a matter of time. I could see my destiny – my life was to vanish, because I couldn't see I had a life anyway.

'Can you read tea leaves?' I asked my 'au pair'.

'No, can you?'

'Yes. Would you like me to read yours?' I was hopeful to make some change in the order of parental guidance. Someone had left a used coffee mug on the table. 'We could pretend the cup is yours.' I pushed the discoloured mug towards her. I already had my own coffee mug. It didn't seem to matter that my beverage wasn't tea. I mean, who would really care in a psych hospital? It was only a matter of fun.

'Okay,' the nurse said.

She's got courage. Should I say something really horrible like she's going to die a terrible death? But then she's living a life of hell anyway. Who would want to work here?

'It's okay. I'll do mine instead,' I said. *I still have compassion.*

'Yes, I'd like to hear your ideas,' she said.

I looked closely into my coffee mug. 'I can see myself in a desert and I'm walking and I'm dying. I don't have any water.'

I looked up and saw another patient who was sitting at another table staring at us. He had long blond and black hair – he looked like Alice Cooper on a really good day.

'You've only seen a mirage,' he said and laughed. 'It happens when you're out in the desert and you don't have any water.'

'Yes, you're very intelligent, Stephen,' the nurse said.

How patronising, even if he does look stupid. I thought my metaphor of myself dying was fairly explicit, hoping she would get the point, but it seemed that one went over her head. I felt my intelligence was being syphoned out of my ears, literally. I knew I couldn't have a conversation based on anything related to joy or happiness. It was just too hard to give – to make people happy, to make them feel better. I just couldn't give any more. *If I'm supposedly psychotic or delusional, well, they must think I am if I'm in here. Perhaps I could pretend I'm not here.*

After tea, I went to the music room, to sit and listen to the stereo. The music room was another area which had a long table, surrounded again by plastic chairs. It had a stereo system on a bench. I had brought some tapes with me and thought it would be a good way to while away some time.

Stephen followed me. I was sitting on the carpet listening to Paul Simon.

'You have to get out of here. This is a sexual molesters' ward. I know the law and the system. You have to beat them at their own game.'

I wondered if Stephen was a sexual molester and if he knew how to get out, then why was he still here?

'It's the only way you'll ever leave,' he said.

'What the hell are you talking about?' Although I didn't think I was going to get a rational response.

'You'll have to put your case in writing.'

'Sounds like you're running for parliament,' I said. *Pity you're not a lawyer.*

'Beware of what you say and if you laugh when no one is in earshot then they'll think you're mad, okay?'

I didn't need him to tell me that.

Before bedtime, I decided to ring my mother. I went to the red phone near the pool table and found some coins in the zippered part of my backpack. I placed the coins into the machine and rang her number. I heard the ringing and then my mother's voice.

'Hello, Mum. It's Gardenia. Can I come home now?

'Oh, no, you can't.'

A direct answer to a direct question.

'What do you mean I can't come home? Why not?'

'It's that you just can't. I'm sorry.'

God, what do I have to do?

I hung up – there wasn't much to talk about.

The au pair that I had compassion for came up to me. 'You're not feeling well. What's happening, Gardenia?'

'I don't want to be a bother. I'm not well that's all. I'm scared I'm going to die.'

'Are your voices telling you that?'

I looked at her and wished I had not said anything. 'I don't hear voices, okay?'

Thank God it was near bedtime and after taking my medication I went up to the sleeping quarters. I had the same room but this time I had a roommate. She was a funny thing, not able to speak English. We did try to communicate but it was impossible. Also I was too stressed to try and I wasn't up to having a chatty discussion even if it had been possible. I was afraid of her and the type of illness she was obviously going through – this I noticed by her capacity to scream in another language.

I ended up placing all my clothes under my bed. I was scared of people pinching things. I wanted to keep something of my own. I knew that the other patients wandered in and out of the rooms. *Can I trust them, people who are unfit to live in the community?*

The strong medication was making me tired – I was relieved I had made it through another day. I heard noise from outside my door, people shouting, screaming. I knew my roommate was crying. Slowly the noise lessened. The cries were diminishing in sound, until everything was silent.

I was still tired in the mornings and the nurses had to pry me out of bed and hold me as they literally dragged me to the showers. I think my looks had significantly deteriorated. I made sure I washed myself and brushed my teeth. I brushed my hair, although it had grown somewhat – it was out of control, a mass of thick curly red hair.

It's okay, I repeated over and over to myself. Even this declaration made me think I was mad, to have a conversation with myself. *It's just my internalised voice in my mind. I'm not hearing voices. Don't we all have loud thoughts in our mind?*

I looked at my eyes in the mirror – they were black like huge dark ink spots. I looked like a mad clown. *It's just a sequence of ideas I'm responding to. My reality is my perception, isn't it?*

I looked in the mirror and could see the doorway behind and this doorway led into another doorway and so on until infinity. I was caught in a time warp. I was lost in dimensions. *Which door do I open? But they're all open. Am I from the past or the present? You can't divide them – it's all one. They're all locked in together – it's all related.*

After three weeks, it was apparent that I was depressed. They stated that I had to undergo another treatment. The physical examination before the treatment noted that I was alert and orientated, cooperative and had visual acuity and muscle tone and power. The doctor tested all the appropriate reflexes with the rubber tool on my elbows and legs and knees. My reflexes were normal and my chest was clear and blood pressure and body temperature were all normal. He examined my breasts and abdomen to make sure there weren't any masses. I had hoped he would notice my hands and arms and the continual tremor. I was worried too about my irregular period and wondered why they weren't investigating this abnormality. Even though I did mention it, there was nothing more said.

I was deemed physically fit for the procedure and I had to sign the consent form to state that they were not liable for anything wrong that might occur.

The procedure was electroconvulsive treatment. I had to be strapped down. The ECT is actually a short epileptic fit. I was given an anaesthetic and the electrodes were placed on my head and tied to another machine.

No one told me anything about the process – what would happen and why it was necessary. I suppose they just thought I was not fit to understand. I had to sign all the legal consent forms for treatment due to the risks involved. My confusion and anxieties had trebled so, not understanding anything of ECT, the event was the most terrifying thing I had ever experienced.

I saw doctors and nurses surrounding me and my hope was that if I died it would not be painful. I imagined the doctor was Paul Simon – it was the only comfort left to me.

Afterwards, as I slowly became conscious, I asked the nurse, 'Is there smoke coming out of my ears?' I suppose there was an association – an appropriate response to having electrodes attached to your head.

I had two weeks of ECT, every second day. The procedure reaffirmed my own self-belief that I was going mad. *I think they'd treat their pet animals better than this.*

I paced up and down hallways in the hospital. I told them that I wanted to go home. I had no idea of what was going on and that the measure of my insanity was bounded by the walls they had me in. *If I mistrust my own mind, then how can I know what I'm thinking is right? If I'm not thinking right, then isn't it best not to talk? They know I'm not insane, don't they? I mean I'm not doing anything bad, am I?*

'Don't you realise I'm living in hell and I can't take it any more?' I screamed out to the other patients and nurses in the ward.

'I don't like her, she's upsetting me,' said an older woman sitting on the couch.

'She's been sitting there all day,' I said. 'I haven't been talking all the time. Do you think I can just sit here all day and night without talking? When am I allowed to talk? Only when you want me to? Then when I want to say what I really feel, then it's not good enough, I can't talk.' *I've just said a lot of senseless rubbish.*

134

'I killed my baby.' I could tell that sent shock waves through the house. *That's why I'm here, isn't it? They're keeping me a prisoner because of that. I'm okay. It will be all right.*

I left the dining area and went to the music room. I sat on the carpet with my back against the wall. I was listening to Simon and Garfunkel – the sounds of silence. *How apt.*

My concentration wasn't very good and my thoughts were getting mixed up. I had the diary my mother gave me and decided to write her a letter.

Dear Mum,
    I'm okay, but I couldn't help having to leave the baby but she will be all right. Now you are looking after her. Don't worry, she will forgive you. She loves you very much.
    I'm sorry.
    Gardenia

'I thought my mother was going to visit me,' I sang out to the nurse who was walking past. She stopped and looked at me and then walked on.

'Where's my mother?' I sang out. 'She's not well. Is she okay? No one's going to kill her, are they?'

I felt so agitated that I danced to alleviate the muscular cramp – my body was in agony. I danced to Paul Simon's 'Diamonds on the soles of her shoes'. I thought he was singing about me. The release of muscular agony diminished as I spiralled around the room. I knew the nurses looked in on me every now and then, trying to see if I was acting accordingly. I didn't care.

The Middle Eastern man came into the music room. I looked at him and he looked at me. I knew what he was thinking. Obviously he wanted sex. I was right. He pulled down the fly of his pants and pulled out his ugly little penis.

I showed him my breasts. 'Like that?' I said. 'How do you like being flashed at, eh? Oh, your genitals are lovely, you better watch out – all the girls will be after you.'

A nurse poked her head around the door. She saw what was happening

'Come on, Paul, come with me please, and Gardenia, I want you to go to the nurses' station now.'

I obeyed.

'Excuse me, I'm important, I'm needed here urgently,' I said, rapping on the glass window of the nurses' office.

The two nurses on duty looked at me.

'How are you this lovely day? Guess you're all wondering about me? Don't worry, because I'm good at everything. Sometimes people don't think I'm good at things, but I don't listen to them, do you? I haven't felt this happy in a long time. I love you all. Do I have to take my medication now?'

The nurses gave me more sedatives and then I had to go into a room just adjacent to the nurses' station. It was called the observation room. It was a small rectangular room with a bed and other essential items needed in emergencies – lots of hypodermic needles.

I saw the nurse get a syringe ready. 'What's that for?' I said.

'Just to make sure you're not pregnant.'

'Who would I be having sex with? You don't think I had sex with Paul? Just because I haven't had a menstrual period in months doesn't mean I'm pregnant, you know.'

She wasn't going to listen to me. She just nodded, saying, 'Yes, I understand.' Pacifying me, I suppose.

'Do you remember what just happened?' Nurse prickles said.

Yes I do, but I'm not going to incriminate myself.

'What happened with Paul?' she said.

'I have no idea what you're talking about.' I thought that was the best answer.

'You know if you do that again, you won't be able to go on leave for the day – to go out with your mother.'

I just looked at her. I pretended it didn't faze me in the least. Actually I did care very much but I wasn't going to let her know that.

'Sure, no worries.'

I suppose the trauma I was experiencing was beginning to show.

Making inappropriate comments was now a way of life for me. At one point I was so scared I was going to swallow my tongue that I lay on the floor placing one arm out and the other arm behind me, in the coma position. I shouted to them, 'Take me away, take me away.'

I think my fluctuating moods were a response to my agitated mind.

'I know what happens in these places,' I sang out. 'You get killed. Don't you understand, everyone – you're all going to die. They're giving you the drugs to sedate you so you don't have a mind any more. They're going to lock me up forever. I know it's going to happen. You're your thoughts and what you think makes the world.' This was conclusive evidence that I had certainly gone off my rocker but it made sense to me.

As time wore on, I changed my thinking to try and relate my situation to theirs. I could not possibly think they were going to kill me, for if they were, it would have happened. So it was likely that the killers were outside. I don't think it helped listening to the Black Sabbath songs and the Doors' 'There's a killer on the run' on the stereo in the music room.

My fears had now quadrupled, believing my life was now over and I was to be locked in an insane asylum for the rest of my life. *Why am I locked in this place – is it because it's safe to be here? Is it due to people being dangerous out there?*

I paced up and down. I couldn't stop my body from moving acrobatically, in positions I think only a gymnast would know. *Are the doors locked? You have to lock them because they'll kill us.*

At night in bed, before the medication took effect, I would howl like a dog. I kept it up for some time. It was like a release, a purging of grief.

It was usual now in the mornings when I'd woken up to see my pants covered in faeces. I had now developed incontinence.

During the next few days, I continued to express my mind and the horrors I was experiencing. Sometimes I felt it was imperative to take all my clothes off. 'I've got to get these clothes off, they just don't fit.' I started undressing.

I felt I knew I was doing something wrong. I stopped and looked about me. I saw a nurse coming towards me.

'It's okay. I'm putting them back on. I won't do it again.'

I would sit near the telephone during the day. I was scared that it would ring. If it did, it would be my mother and that would only mean one thing. She was dead. Also, I was afraid that if it did ring, I would have to answer it, and what would happen then? I couldn't communicate.

My paranoia about my circumstances was on a grand scale. *I know the nurses are looking at me and I wonder if they know what I'm thinking. Perhaps they can read my thoughts and if they can, then they'll know I'm mad. Are they telling the doctor what I'm doing?*

Often I would sit looking out of the window. I could see the branches and leaves of the various native gum trees swaying with the wind. I could see vacant wooden benches placed in and around the smaller native bushes. It gave an isolated impression. I could have been in the countryside and the only inhabitants were birds, small lizards and other animals. I wondered how I could draw the trees. I mimicked quick hand gestures with a pretend pencil. I was producing scribbled, patterned lines. It was then that I knew what I had to do – I felt a sense of hope. I was going to go home.

The chance came later that evening. I heard a loud ringing reverberate inside the day room. It was a fire drill and the nurses rounded up the patients like cattle and we all stood outside on a patch of green lawn. I had little hope of ever returning to my home so, as the emergency procedure was taking place, I made up my mind to run as fast as I could go, away from Felixstowe. I knew my way home – I had lived in this city all my life.

I ran out into the night, down the footpath and towards the main road. I didn't look behind me – I was too concerned that they would follow, so my speed was essential. The cool air was refreshing and I felt like Lassie in an old movie, able to sense my way home. The thought of this made me feel better – like it was a strong connection to something that was good. It appeased my fearful and petrified mind, it was a liberating force. *I have an important purpose – it's the right thing for me to do or perhaps I'm having a near-death experience and I'll soon be in heaven.*

The hospital was in North Fitzroy, near the city. I got on a tram at

Brunswick Street. I had forgotten about the fare and as I sat down I hoped no one would ask me to pay, because I didn't have any money. I watched out the window, the retail shops going past, and then I noticed that the driver was looking at me. He called out and said I had to pay for a ticket. I told him I couldn't pay as I didn't have any money, to which he replied, 'God help us all.'

The tram took me into the city and then to the outer western suburbs towards the West Gate Bridge. I reasoned how far I had gone and the direction I was heading. When the tram turned to the south, I decided it would be best to get off, as my home was not far away.

I still had a long walk ahead of me to get to my suburb, Spotswood. I passed the weatherboard houses. I could just make out their exteriors in the moonlight – shades of blue, pink and green, colours I had never noticed before. There were numerous trees in this area and small gardens. I had to cross a large park; it was isolated, ominous. I could see the orchard of olive trees with their trunks bent and immovable – like ghosts. I quickly walked on. I was jumpy, frightened of the dark. The street lights were few and far between and up ahead I saw a car parked on the side of the road. I saw the passenger door open. I remembered the time when I was young and a man tried to force me into his car. I was able to fight my way free. Perhaps I could do it again?

I could be murdered.

I boldly walked past the car. *It won't take me long, my home isn't far away – I'll be there soon.*

The footpath shadows were getting larger and I tried to tell myself that it was only my imagination. My senses were acute and I could sense people watching me, hiding in the foliage, ready to jump out. I kept turning my head around, expecting a stranger. I didn't know if I was screaming but it felt like I was.

I could see flowers on the side of the road and I remembered planting roses in the garden at home when I was younger. I remembered my father showing me the stars pointing to the night sky and saying, 'That's the Milky Way.' I remembered him saying, 'Never lose faith in yourself.' I looked up to the bright night sky – its dark expanse was proliferated with tiny white sparkles.

I could feel my feet throbbing as if I was treading on broken pieces of glass.

My initial enthusiasm had dwindled. I was tired and thirsty. I saw in front of me a major intersection; it was Halls Road. I recognised the landmarks – McDonald's and Hungry Jack's. *I'm nearly there.*

I was relieved to see my childhood home. It was a simple red-brick structure with a gravelled pathway, garden beds at the front and side. At the front, there was an arch with climbing roses. It was like a cottage garden, with succulents, native trees and bushes. I sat on the front bench under the veranda and contemplated my situation.

When I knocked on the door, I expected my mother to be surprised.

'Gardenia, what have you done now?' she said.

Well, that's a great welcome.

'The police are after you, do you realise that? They've been ringing me.'

I walked in and poured myself a glass of water from the sink. I guzzled the liquid and then refilled it again.

'I'm never going back there, do you hear?' I looked at my mother's face. It was lined and her eyes were small dark spots. I could see that I was doing her an injustice. She didn't have to suffer because of me.

'Okay, but I'll ring them and let them know you're all right,' she said.

I could tell that my mother knew the situation as well as I did. When dealing with authority, you have to obey their requests. She would have loved me to stay at home, I knew that, but could she defy their rules and regulations? I considered that the only alternative I had was to go back and face the consequences.

I heard my mother speaking to the hospital on the phone.

'Yes, she'll come right back. We'll have some tea and then, yes, in another hour.'

I had been placed on the missing persons list and when I came back to the ward, I knew they were not pleased by my actions. I was not pleased to be back again – I was angry at the injustice of it all.

'There are some limitations to cruelty,' I shouted at the nurses gathered around me as they forced me to take my medication. I had no idea they had a form of punishment in mind.

In their minds, I had absconded and therefore I had to be detained in a secure ward. They obviously thought I was psychotic and a danger to myself and others. I think they just didn't like the fact that I walked home.

Even though the secure ward was in another part of the hospital grounds, I still had to have a police escort. I sat in the back seat of a car between two men in dark suits, 'security officers'. I didn't know at the time they were guards, because my situation was too confusing. I thought they were henchmen and I had just been given the death penalty. I wondered if I was in a movie about the French Revolution and was I an aristocrat, waiting for judgement. *Hanging. Anything's possible.*

'My feet hurt. I'll need some shoes, if we're going to see all the art galleries,' I said. I was lost in another fantasy – this reality was too frightening.

In the dark, with only a few lights to demarcate the area, I saw the high-security hospital – it had a bleak and forbidding countenance.

I signed more papers relating to my detainment. I wondered why I had to sign the forms. *Doesn't one have to be coherent or mentally aware of what they are signing? But in their minds I'm psychotic.*

I said I was a lawyer – it was an adequate response because there were so many forms to sign. It was my way of understanding my situation, because I had lost all contact with my former life. I now lived in an abusive and intolerant system.

*

```
Nursing summary and nursing intervention
Date: 21st January
Thought disorder: states she feels confused.
Poor appetite, weight loss. Observe food and fluid
intake.
Auditory hallucinations: likelihood of acting in
response to her altered perception. Observe auditory
```

hallucinations and her desire of acting on them
Risk of absconding behaviour monitor to minimise risk.
Tendency to disinhibition: stripping herself.
Continues to need constant supervision to limit her
bizarre behaviour; disturbing other patients.
Orientate and reassure patient.
Sleep chart use of prn medication.
Problems remain the same.

Inpatient records
Date: 21st January
Doctor Grimshaw

Gardenia Baxter
Looseness of association: Gardenia says it is 30th of
December 1986 when it is 1st of January 1987.
Has a 'passivity phenomena' with thought broadcasting
insertion. Has ideas of reference and confusion of
self. As part of her admission it was recommended that
she should be detained.
Schizophrenia with acute relapse.
Her appearance is neat and appropriately dressed.
Reactive with perception intact. Cognition good;
insight good; rapport good. The increase in fluphenazine
would be the reason for her now calming affect.
Paranoid; given extra dosages. Gardenia states 'she
feels threatened by being in here afraid that we are
out to get her'.
Nurses and staff report that 'she is panicky and is
running around'.
Also noted that she said to another patient 'just
listen to the music'.
Gardenia appears to be somewhat muddled after ECT and
spends a lot of time wandering.
She is grossly thought-disordered and paranoid and
the increased dosages had little effect as she is
disorganised with thought blocking and fear of being
killed; she is running from imaginary assailants.
Mother expressed a basic understanding of Gardenia's
disorder; mother expresses concern re Gardenia's well
being.

Inpatient records

Date: 30th January
Doctor Grimshaw

Gardenia Baxter
Her behaviour is inappropriate and has tried to
abscond three times.
She is aggressive towards staff.
Requiring time out and medication.
Mother is frustrated and wants to take her home.
Has relapsed on imiprimine; need to change medication.
Commenced chlorpromazine, stelazine and benzotrophine
with some effect.
At seven o'clock this evening Gardenia Baxter not
found to be in unit.
Last seen five minutes to seven. 7.15 p.m. search of
unit. 7.20 p.m. police notified missing person.
Relative notified by nursing supervisor at 7.45 p.m.
Medical officer notified at 7.50 p.m.
At 8.40 p.m. phone call from mother who located
Gardenia at front door step. Says she will stay for
tea and be back after that. To return at 2100 hours.
On return very distraught and delusional screaming
loudly and placed in secure room as attempted to leave
unit again. Mother says she will visit tomorrow.
Gardenia was discharged from open ward to be admitted
to secure ward. She left unit with police escort.
Gardenia Baxter is a security risk and therefore needs
continual observation.

9

Felixstowe Hospital
Referral for admittance to secure ward

Gardenia Baxter
Gardenia Baxter is a twenty one year old woman
experiencing initially schizophrenia. She is currently
undertaking tertiary studies. She has marked depression
symptomology. Has a history of use and abuse of
marijuana, speed and magic mushrooms.
She has paranoia, thought disorder and restlessness.
She has been stripping off her clothes.
Denies any auditory hallucinations but many times
throughout the day becomes distracted and appears to
be listening to something.
Occasionally through the day she cries for no apparent
reason. Also has been observed to be laughing with no
obvious reason.
Has no insight.
Absconding risk.
Potential self harm.
The most distressing feature of Gardenia's distress is
her howling 'in despair'.
Her mother is also very worried.
Given fluphenazine at 800 hours and 1300 hours and 1700
hours.
We are concerned that she does not appreciate the need
for her treatment due to impaired insight.

*

I was led into an area and I watched the doors being locked behind me.
They took me to a desk where I had to sign forms.

'You know I'm a lawyer,' I said.

There are so many papers to sign – therefore I must be a lawyer.

I did have temporary insight, although this knowledge was sporadic and perplexing, like an abstract dream. I realised at different times that I was locked in some type of secure hospital ward and meaningful ideas would germinate. Saying I was a lawyer, thinking I was somebody else, comforted me. My paranoid thinking had not ceased. I still believed they were going to kill me and to me it was a logical deduction – why else would I be treated this way?

I was then taken to a large room and told to undress. This was an old part of the hospital. It had high ceilings and hard concrete walls. There were two small windows which looked out onto the grounds and black iron bars attached on the outside of the windows. Part of the room had a tiled floor and I noticed two cubicles made of brick without doors attached. The room had no furnishings except one plastic chair where I could place my clothes.

Two male nurses watched me as I took my clothes off. One of the men told me to go into the brick-like cubicle and I crouched in the corner as he sprayed me with a long hose. My body felt the pressure of the cold hard water. After this initial cleansing, they dressed me in men's pyjamas which were placed on me with the buttons at the back. After that, I was led into a cell-like room with a mattress on the floor; the locked door had a small square window.

I could not relate my circumstances to anything I had previously seen or understood, not in a practical sense. I could not rationalise why people would lock me in a prison. I could only connect with my visual memory. I had seen a movie of Jewish people in Nazi Germany. I saw the women and children wandering in a glass prism or cage, screaming as the poisonous gas entered the chamber. In slow motion, I saw them fall to the ground. I wanted to be dead too. I thought they were lucky to have died, because I knew my torture was to continue.

I tried to keep my mind focused on what the time was and how long I had been locked up. It was for at least two days. They brought me in food and drink. I think there was a routine and every two hours they opened the cell door and I was allowed to go to the toilet.

I was told to take the medication. While I was in the cell, I made frequent attempts to get their attention. I screamed but I did not keep it up for long because it hurt my throat. I made ugly and horrific disfiguring faces at the small window, hoping by some miracle they would notice and let me out. My conditions living in this cell made me evaluate my chances of survival. The conclusion that I would not live, or return to my home, was conclusive. I prayed for another chance. The screams I heard from the other locked-up souls made me think I was in some form of hell.

After the second day, I was allowed out of the cell. I walked down a hallway, past the toilet and bathroom areas that were to one side. I was taken to a larger room. The walls were white and the linoleum flooring was white. There weren't any windows. There was a red rubber mat in the corner, and some plastic chairs and a table in the middle of the room. There was a large glass window and behind it I saw men studying me. On the other side of the room against the wall were ten or twelve plastic chairs. Sitting on the chairs were men and I could see their eyes staring at me, devouring every move I made. I felt like a monkey in a cage. I was being evaluated like an anthropologist studies a new primitive species.

Another door led out of this room to a dining area which consisted of four tables, each with four chairs, and a servicing area. A blue line demarcated the two areas – the dining tables and the kitchen. Although they did not tell me, I knew I was not allowed to cross the line. There was another door which led to the outside, where there was a large expanse of lawn, a volleyball net and, surrounding it, a high barbed-wire fence.

I was not alone, as there were two other patients in this ward. I found one patient in particular very disturbing as he continually liked to hover around me and make buzzing noises in my ear. The other man did not have any fingers and I often looked at him knowing I was safe because he could not strangle me.

I worked out quickly who was in charge in relation to the nurses. A tall nurse named Luke held the keys and I called to him often, speaking nicely and saying hello. My hope was that he would see I was a good person – worthy of being allowed my freedom. I think he thought I was making a proposition.

He followed me to the toilet block and proceeded to fondle my breasts. 'Doesn't that make you feel better?' he said.

I knew at the time that I could not say anything – who would believe me?

I spent a month in this ward and mostly in the white room. I would sit at the table and poke my tongue out at the nurses who studied me. Often I would sit in the corner on the rubber mat and cry. In the dining area, I would sometimes jump across the blue line and say 'Boo' then jump back.

There were times when I would make callisthenic-type movements with my body, pushing my arms and legs in various contorted positions. It seemed to relieve some pain I was undergoing. It was an unreal world and nothing made sense.

My mother visited me for fifteen minutes once a day. She would bring me a carton of chocolate milk. We never spoke and I drank the cold liquid hungrily as if it was my only source of survival.

The patient who did not have any fingers was named Frank. He was short with a long straggly beard. Sometimes I wondered if he was one of the seven dwarfs.

We were sitting in the dining area. I didn't look at him while he ate, as I thought it was rude to stare. I never did know how he managed to eat his food.

'They do a good job of the interior decorating, don't they?' he said.

'I feel like I'm a mole or something, in tunnels under the earth,' I said.

'These stone walls have salt damp, that's why they're a dirty grey colour,' said Frank. 'It will all have to be repainted, you know,' he continued.

Obviously, I thought.

'Let's go out and get some fresh air,' he said. 'Come on, I'll show you the church.'

I walked with him down to the end near the barbed-wire fence. I saw before me an expanse of land, punctuated with old buildings. Some of the structures were decaying and were obviously not occupied. The buildings had deteriorated with time, due to lack of maintenance. Their uninhabitable presence, in a vast landscape, made them look odd and disturbing. I felt like I was in a Western, in film studios, where only the fronts of the buildings were seen. They were like a shell, fabricated to make them look real. I could imagine the empty structures, their set design, with actors and cameras telling a story. I imagined the frightening scenes, the stories of patients, their traumatic lives, imprisoned in these ghostly structures.

'See that building, the old one just there?' He pointed.

'Yes,' I said.

'That's the church,' he said.

'It's beautiful, isn't it?' I said, thinking I should show respect. 'It looks old.' Suddenly a burst of sunlight shone through the clouds directly on to my face.

'It's very dramatic, isn't it? It's not too elaborate. I guess you don't want that here. See that elaborate piece of sculptured iron work at the front?' the man said.

'Yes, the cross.' I saw the large symbol of rebirth situated at the top of the decayed building.

'I invented that,' he said. 'That's the main building over there, where all the doctors work. I think royalty used to live there. See all the other buildings.' He pointed to a group of smaller houses that sat on the perimeter of the grounds. 'All the workers or servants lived in those. The government own it now.'

I felt like I was on some macabre tour. He was making sense, except for inventing the cross, but then metaphorically he was living in hell and Christianity was about rebirth – he certainly had a cross to bear.

'See that, the baby bird?' he said.

'The one that's fallen from the nest?' I said.

'In the midst of life there is death. Their small bony bodies will decompose into the earth. It's destiny and eventually we will all die,' he said. 'John Maynard Keynes said in the long term we're all going to die.'

I knew about Keynesian economics and pondered this reality. Sure enough, we were all trying to work out how to manage limited resources, but how can you really estimate the future?

'Isn't it how we live that matters?' I said.

'Let's not talk about that any more. I can't tell you everything, because the CIA are after me. By the way, do you want to be my girlfriend?' he said.

I didn't reply. I wondered how long he had been in the hospital and whether he remembered any of his former life. *He just has a vivid imagination and likes living in a fantastical world. It helps him cope in a scary world. It's like living a slow death in here. How can any of us expect to go back into the community? Or is that required? It's like we're cattle pushed into stuffy caged prisons, without escape. Is this a place of refuge, asylum? Can anyone recover in these conditions?*

We went back to the dining area and the man pointed to the table in the corner.

'See that table there?' he said.

'That one?' I pointed to the white plastic table, but then all the tables looked the same.

'I invented that table but don't tell anyone. They wanted to take the design away from me. I know who shot J.F. Kennedy and that's why the CIA are after me.'

Didn't they already know who shot J.F. Kennedy? Wasn't it Lee Harvey Oswald?

'Do you have any money? I guess not. I'll buy you a cup of coffee, but you have to pay me back, okay?' he said.

'Sure,' I said. I wasn't afraid of him. I knew he enjoyed my company and even if he didn't make sense, there wasn't really a lot I could do about it.

He went up to the counter and asked the nurse for two cups of coffee.

'Just a minute. I'll bring them to your table,' she said.

We sat there, both of us staring into space.

'We have to wait here,' he said. 'It's time for our appointment and they'll see us soon.'

'Okay,' I said. At least we were having a conversation and it was the first time in ages I had been able to connect with someone.

'See those framed pieces of paper – that means they're qualified.'

He pointed to the noticeboard that hung on the wall. Posters or papers were pinned to it. I thought it might have been the nurses' roster duties. *Should I ask what time they're expecting us? Perhaps they've forgotten about our appointment?*

In the distance, I could hear screaming. I wondered if humans were making that noise, or could it be the wheels of motor vehicles? It was an anguished cry, like a wail. I knew it wasn't idiots driving and screeching their tyres.

As part of my detainment in a locked award, I was to undergo another course of ECT. I had to sign the consent form again, allowing them to perform this minor surgery, to make sure that if anything went wrong, the hospital was not responsible.

I'm not sure if it was because I participated in a game of volleyball with the nurses that I was discharged from the secure ward. Perhaps they presumed I was coherent enough, or that the medication might have contributed to my improvement. I signed more papers and was transferred by police escort once more to my previous ward

As I was leaving the building, a nurse said something enigmatic to me. 'Remember why you came here?'

I didn't understand the reason. It was the first occasion a nurse had spoken to me on a person-to-person basis in all that time.

I tried to have a sense of humour during this time because I knew that things could not get any worse. During my stay I understood a poignant idea and I have never forgotten it. I realised that it didn't matter where I was, or in what circumstances I found myself, I still had a form of control. I still had my mind and, considering what I had been through, how I had been treated, I had survived. This sense of self gave me a source of power. I knew then that whatever medication they forced me to take or how barbaric their medical science was, they could not take away my humanity. This was expressed through my character and my personality. Ironically, in facing this primeval fear of insanity and death, I understood my real identity. I was able to close the gates on all that was superficial, the elements of assumptions – the external world. My mind was the only thing left and I was no longer afraid of that.

*

Inpatient records
Felixstowe Hospital
Secure Ward
Doctor Reddon

Gardenia Baxter
Date 28th February.

Summary
Gardenia Baxter has been experiencing auditory and
visual hallucinations and displaying grandiose
delusions.
'I'm a lawyer.'
Thought disorder - fearful and paranoid.
'Someone's trying or going to kill me.'
Placed in seclusion for first two nights of her
admission - she was disturbing other patients.
She has been an absconding risk and has remained in
dressing gown and pyjamas.
Her affect is now reactive and appropriate. Slight
confusion is still evident on occasions but she is now
showing some insight and realises she is confused.
Inappropriate behaviour such as undressing and
propositioning male staff has not been evident in the
last 24 hours.
The side effect of increasing medication of fluphenazine
has exacerbated her anxiety although she is more
settled and improving. We see that depression and
anxiety will need to be more specifically treated.
She has related in quiet cooperative manner accepting
of her need for continued inpatient care in a closed
setting. She can be transferred back to open ward.

10

After my time in the seclusion ward, I spent another four months in the open unit. My health deteriorated during this time and my depression continued. I was not eating and I continued to have regular enemas, once a week. They saw my vomiting in the mornings as a symptom of pregnancy and I had to undergo more tests. My medication was continually being changed. I could tell this by the varying colours of the tablets and the amount. I was also having numerous blood tests and was given another course of ECT treatment. My condition had not improved with their treatments. Perhaps it was not due to an organic illness, but psychological.

When the nurses asked me questions, I replied with the only subject I could understand – my past and memories of movies I had seen. I did not have the strength now to carry out a conversation or even to feel anger. At times I would pray to God, to sense his presence, to find an answer.

I was sitting in the television area, looking out the window, when one of the nurses came up and sat down beside me.

'That's nice,' she said.

I had taken a small cane basket from the craft room. I had sewn a piece of cloth on the inside as a lining. I was going to place my brush and soap in it, to have it on my dressing table in my room.

'I can't talk because I must have a tooth pulled and I can't go to the toilet,' I said.

The nurse hesitated before she spoke. 'Why can't you go to the toilet, Gardenia?'

'Because I can't urinate,' I said.

'Have you tried running water? That sometimes helps.'

'I've tried everything, even having a bath. I haven't been for hours and my bladder hurts.'

'I see.'

I was still feeling very uncomfortable when my mother came to visit.

'How are you today, Gardenia?' She always gave me a big beaming smile.

'Not too good. I can't urinate.'

'Have you told the nurses?' she said.

'Yes.'

'How long has it been since you last went to the toilet?'

'Last night. I'm really in pain now. I can hardly walk. Can you help me? It's getting worse.'

'I'll talk to a nurse.'

My mother forced them to take action and I was given a catheter. The nurses commented on how amazing it was to have so much fluid in my bladder.

I had another catheter the next week due to fluid retention. I had no idea it was due to the effects of medication. I thought it was just another sign of my mental illness. My irrational thoughts were making my body malfunction.

I spent the next four months waiting in the open ward, hoping for my release. Much of my time was taken up by dancing in the music room, another carpeted area that had a stereo player. It seemed not many of the other patients liked this room, so I spent as much time in there as I could. It helped me to dance, because my muscles were rigid like sticks and I needed to flex them to make myself comfortable. It was agonising to have continual cramp and a restlessness that wouldn't go away. Then there were times when my exhaustion was overpowering. I was not allowed to go to my bedroom, and the couches in the day room were always taken, so I would lie in the observation room, just for some peace and quiet.

My appetite had decreased and I was now skin and bone, the weight of a large dog, fifty-two kilos. I was tall, one hundred and sixty-eight centimetres in height. By this time, I understood the seriousness of my situation. I had to compromise to get their help now, for my survival. I agreed with them saying I was paranoid, that I was scared and I was hearing voices. I had regressed now to the point of being a child. When my mother visited me, I would cry. The social worker recommended that my mother should not visit because of this response. I think it was at this time that my mother decided to take me home. She knew I was not going to get better in this hospital, so I was allowed trial leave. Was I no longer a threat to them any more, because I agreed with their diagnosis and symptoms? Or did they think their job was finished, sedating me to the point of being a walking vegetable?

My mother stood by my side and gently took me by the hand and led me away from the confines of Felixstowe. I had not seen a doctor while I was an inpatient. My treatment was based on nurses' observation.

There were conditions attached to my leaving hospital. I had to return each week to be monitored and assessed. To have consultations with the duty doctor and to undergo more blood tests with lithium and carbamazepine levels. Also I had to be admitted again if my mother needed respite.

The thought of home, having a stabilised environment and a different life, gave me hope.

*

Outpatient records
Doctor Grimshaw

Gardenia Baxter
Date: 30th June

States she feels confused but doesn't know why.
States she has occasional hallucinations. Still
continues to have fears about dying and being killed.
Occasionally uses threatening voice and facial
expression.
Continuing looseness of association and thought
blocking. Sometimes stares upwards and when questioned,
states she 'can see her father up there'. Is it visual
hallucinations?
She remains psychotic and agitated in behaviour. Also
appears to be reacting from messages from radio at

times. Continues to have frustrated, angry and teary outbursts but settles. Her minimal integration with staff and other patients is because 'other patients torment me'.

Wants her mother to come and see her. Says her mother doesn't understand her and doesn't care about her and she wants to die. Episodes of crying during the day and is frightened her mother is in danger, that someone will kill her. She has tearful episodes when Mother visits and appears to be responding to voices at this time as she wants reassurance from Mother. She requires supervision with meals to ensure adequate diet intake. She manages to eat most of her meals with reassurance. Although her eating and fluids has diminished considerably, when Mother visited she helped herself to food and drink!!!

Still remains unsettled, unable to sit for any length of time. She walks the corridors and wanders around the unit. She listens to her walkman looking confused and lost. Said she wanted to speak to a patient and at night was found in his room and promptly put back to bed. Her mental state still remains poor requiring close supervision. Although she is cooperative with staff still needs to be monitored to prevent her from wandering off.

She admits quite correctly that she needs treatment but I wonder if she is not playing into a role now, perhaps covering up psychotic thoughts.

Gardenia is becoming more positive in her outlook. Seems more relaxed and general behaviour is better. She laughs spontaneously in appropriate settings. Has been doing craftwork and wants to start painting but has poor concentration span. She paints only for a limited time and has a distant effect. She states 'I prefer listening to music rather than sitting in silence'. There is a possibility of thought broadcasting, as she stated that 'the nurse knows what I am thinking.'

She has been out during day with Mother. They caught a bus to riverside and watched the ducks. She was quite teary on return, sad and wants to go home.

I have given information to Mother regarding Gardenia's illness.

Mother wants Gardenia home so have agreed to trial
leave. On condition that Gardenia comes back once a
week for continued assessment.
Have increased chlorpromazine medication but still
requires fluphenazine prn. To commence haloperidol
in addition to regular medication and to increase
regularity of lorazepam.
To continue with temazepam during day.

Signed
Doctor Grimshaw

11

I returned to Felixstowe as an outpatient and in the next seven years I was regularly seen every two weeks during this period. Doctor Grimshaw was the first of many student doctors I was to see during this time. They were different only in person but not in ideas.

During those years, I tried to tell the doctors that I did not suffer from a mental illness. Their diagnosis was schizo-affective disorder. I knew I was not experiencing hallucinations but my 'diagnosis' was irrelevant. I looked up the definition in a current dictionary and the term meant I was suffering from a psychotic illness with additional mood disorder. I had to agree with their ideas, knowing the possible consequences, the seclusion ward. I continued to be afraid of the hospital and the continuing analyses.

I learnt very quickly after my hospitalisation to compromise with the mental health system. I couldn't win the war to change my diagnosis, because that was not an option. I learnt to adapt, trying to understand their theories, rules and ideas. I tried to understand the different types of medication and how to react to such drugs. Lithium for mood swings, the antidepressants for depression, obviously, and the antipsychotics for delusional thinking. Sadly, I believed that everything I thought was irrational in some way. Even a logical idea had some ulterior paranoid motive. Consequently I took benzodiazepines, the minor tranquillisers, to quell my anxieties in this regard.

I tried to stay positive when talking to the doctors, expressing my anxiety and depression in a way that didn't imply a 'weird' mind. I understood that the definition of anxiety meant worry or fear, and depression was related to feeling sad. These symptoms I could honestly say I had, and I tried my best to answer their questions and describe my thoughts in relation to my prevalent but speculative emotions. Schizophrenia held too many negative connotations. It was a prognosis that created a future of doubt and uncertainty for me. The ongoing medication, the repeated jury-style interviews, the monthly blood tests and the psychological impact of thinking myself insane held little prospect for a happy life. I had felt forced or coerced to agree with the doctors' plans. I realised that the definitions of mental illness were created by theoreticians or researchers. I wondered if their minds were sick.

My lack of self-confidence and submissiveness was evident in such basic things as asking my mother for permission to have a shower. The prescription of temazepam, sleeping tablets, was a godsend. I took them throughout the day. I slept off and on for three years. The induced rest was curative. It helped me to block out recent memories of Felixstowe, distancing me from the hospital trauma.

My mother understood this and helped me. She was my counsellor who relieved my fears. I know she saved my life. I didn't have to thank God for this 'miracle'. It was my mother who deserves the gratitude. She understood the hospital's conditions had upset me more than any significant mental disorder.

I wanted to eventually discontinue my fortnightly analyses in the interviewing room and the medications, but how to do that was another question. I certainly didn't tell them I was taking sleeping tablets during the day, but they weren't aware I was taking more than usual.

After three years of sleeping, I returned to study part-time at university. It was something I had to do to prove my sanity, to believe in myself. Although I still had many difficulties with poor concentration and social anxiety, I made a concerted effort. With the large amounts of tranquillisers in my body, I had to learn to read and write again. I had to understand the basic constructs in the use of sentences, how to logically make an argument, and my memory was not good, so it was hard going to understand the lectures. I wondered if it was socially permissible to do a university course and have a mental illness. I didn't tell the lecturers I had a schizo-affective disorder because I didn't need the added negativity. I was sure they wouldn't see me in a positive manner. I think my tutors understood my anxieties because they never asked me to speak publicly about my research, which I appreciated. They passed my essays with the recurrent report that my ideas were 'novel'. A nice way of saying I had original ideas but application of the technical information was not considered. In my last year of university, I failed a subject. It was a difficult anthropology area dealing with African regional cults. My lecturer told me I had written senseless ideas and needed to go back and learn to write. I did receive high marks in a first year subject related to art history and theory. However, I took his criticism seriously and I did not go back to my studies.

I had another appointment with a new duty doctor at Felixstowe. I had made my mind up that this would be the last time. I would not be going back.

'Hello, Gardenia. I'm Doctor Tether. How are you today?'

He had blond wavy hair and a moustache. He reminded me of a character who should have been in a Starsky and Hutch film in the 70s.

'Yes, well, I'm okay. I've been going to courses, like always,' I said.

'And how are your thoughts?'

'I'm concentrating a bit better,' I said. *I have to reaffirm my belief in myself somehow?* 'I think the abortion was the reason for my illness,' I said. It was my attempt to rationalise their diagnosis.

His eyes were blue and vacant-looking. I don't think he liked my manner. He was a clinical diagnostician and he had already made up his mind and didn't like others to tell him otherwise.

'And what have you been doing?'

'My mother and I catch buses together. We go out for coffee or grocery shopping. Sometimes we just go for a walk.'

I thought about telling him of how I still tripped on the pavement. *He won't listen anyway.*

'It's a type of desensitisation, trying to do practical physical things, to overcome my anxieties. It helps with my panic attacks because that leads to anxiety and then depression then low self-esteem, then circling back to social anxiety, then agoraphobia.' *God, that was a mouthful.*

He didn't respond. I watched him writing his notes. I was not looking forward to telling him I was not coming back. *Do I have the courage?*

'I see you didn't want to be involved in the rehabilitation programme. Why?'

The truth was that I wanted something better for myself. I did not want to go backwards, to learn basic life skills, to be patronised. Could I tell him that? They still didn't understand that I had been at university in the last two years. I wondered if they had even written it in their reports.

'I'm just not ready,' I said. 'I get depressed and feel a failure. I don't think people like me.' I looked at my hands and I could see a slight tremor. *Should I tell him about the enemas I'm still having at the hospital or that I'm still only having two periods a year? I don't think it's worth it. Can I tell him about my jerky movements, or agitation? Would he like to know about my excess saliva and my constant drooling? He already knows all that and even if I do explain it to him, he'll only assume I'm psychotic again.*

'You wanted to be placed on a disability pension, is that right?' he said.

I nodded. It was the last thing I wanted but the social worker had other ideas. 'I suppose it's the only viable alternative, given my illness. I suppose you still think I have a mental illness even though I'm going to university?' *I wonder how he'll approach that one.*

'It's in remission,' he said.

How can I have a psychotic disorder one day and not the next?

'The medication has helped,' he continued.

It didn't in the first place. Getting away from this institution has made me better.

'Do you know what I was studying at university and are you interested?' I smiled and laughed.

By his expression I could see he was questioning my audacity to even ask him such a question?

'No. Do tell,' he said.

'Second year anthropology subjects – myth, ritual and religion and peasantry rebellion,' I said. 'Also I studied an architecture subject.' I didn't want to tell him I had failed a third year topic.

'Did you enjoy it?' he said.

'I'm having some time off at the moment, but I'm enjoying my artwork. Did you know I received two awards this year for my drawings?' I said.

'No, really?'

He doesn't look interested. Am I boring him?

'I received a distinction for an essay about propaganda,' I continued.

'Really?'

Well, he doesn't have much to say, does he? So does he still think I'm deranged?

'I don't think the carbamazepine is doing that much for me,' I said. 'It makes me tired and I can't concentrate.' I was afraid of continued epileptic fits and asking to decrease tablets wasn't an offence. 'Also I'd like a smaller dose of the perphenazine and I'd like to stop the lithium.' I felt like I was in a corner shop ordering my lunch. It had taken me six years to gain the courage to say that.

Doesn't he understand that I need to have some dignity and self-respect? I want a quality of life. Is that too much too ask? I really don't know why I bother but then I have little choice. Coming to this place week after week is like going to court. I wonder what the verdict will be today – life sentence? This illness is only relevant while I'm in this interview room. What is schizo-affective disorder anyway?

They never did give me an answer, not a specific one. It was as if the general label was enough, but that didn't help me to understand. I wondered about the role of these professionals and their actions or inclinations. I thought the psychiatrist's role was to clarify or explain the reason for a person's problem.

'How do you feel now about your time in hospital, then?' he asked.

'It was an abandonment of love,' I said. *Does he want me to explain to him what's wrong with me?*

'I'm not coming back here, you know.'

'What do you mean, Gardenia?'

'I'm not coming back to Felixstowe again to see you.'

'I don't think that's a very good idea.'

'Why? Because you think I'll go stark raving mad?'

'No, I didn't say that.'

No, you didn't have to.

'I have to keep on taking your pills but I'm the one who's doing all the work, not your chemicals,' I said.

'Don't make me get forceful with you, Gardenia. You come here on a voluntary basis.'

'I've had it, this is enough. I can't take it any more. I have not got schizophrenia and I'm not coming back, got it?'

I didn't wait for his reply. I walked out of the interview room and out into the light. I was not going back there and I was going to make sure of it.

I knew after leaving Felixstowe that I would still need to see a doctor. The medication was another thing. Withdrawal from mind-altering drugs would not be easy. Also, if they had it in mind to detain me, I would just say I was seeing another psychiatrist. That was my only alternative as I did not have the strength to combat such a powerful system.

I came home and wondered what my mother's response would be.

'What did the doctor say? He rang me and said you were angry and stormed out. He said you weren't going back there.' She looked alarmed and I was sorry for her.

'Oh yes, and what else did he say?'

'He said that if I think you're doing something strange or your behaviour's out of the ordinary, to take you back there for hospitalisation.'

'Oh yes, and have you ever seen me do something strange or out of the ordinary?'

'No, Gardenia, I've never seen you like that. I've never agreed with them and their ideas. I don't think you have schizophrenia and I think they've made a very big mistake.'

'Thanks, Mum.'

'I said to him that the medications have made you worse and it was a good thing that you were leaving and I hung up on him. What are you going to do now, Gardenia?'

Her strength and dominant opinion did not make me feel better, although it gave me some relief. I had to work out the next step. I was angry that I had to challenge a medical system, to find other alternatives, to remedy their misconduct.

'I'm going to see a private psychiatrist.'

I wondered why my mother had not taken me to a private psychiatrist. Perhaps she had tried, or was it about the money? Maybe she was waiting for me to act.

'Who are you going to see?' she said.

'I'll look for one in the phone book.' *Anyone would be better than those doctors at Felixstowe.*

'Did you tell him how well you are?'

'I said I was getting better and that I use a desensitisation process.'

'What did he say about that?'

'Nothing.' I wondered if she was in my shoes how she would react. 'If you had a bad memory, would you think you had an illness?'

'No, of course not. Everyone forgets sometimes,' she said.

'Well, I know you go off the track sometimes, Mum, but it doesn't mean you're a nut, does it?' I saw her face and I realised I had hurt her. 'No, I'm just joking, Mum.'

God, she's more sensitive than I am and that's saying something.

'I can see your point, Gardenia.'

Thank God someone does.

*

Outpatient's records
Doctor Tether

Gardenia Baxter
A psychotic disorder is still prevalent with symptoms of thought blocking. Doesn't get to the point quickly, is circular.
She is still preoccupied with her long hospital stay and has issues about her admission. This is natural as it is part of her adjustment back into society.

She is bright-eyed and reactive but her attempts to be friendly are a bit too over-familiar. She is an extremely sensitive person.

Angry outburst. States she is not coming back for consultation. Rang mother and told her if she behaves strangely to have her admitted.

Current medication is…

500 mg Lithium morning and night
Perphenazine 8mg tds 16mg nocte and prn
Benztropine 2mg morning and night.
Temazepam 10-20 mg nocte at night.
Lorazepam 1mg prn
Prothiadin 150mg at night.

Signed
Doctor Tether

12

To say that Kensington Clinic was different to Felixstowe would be an understatement. I was once more in the garden at the clinic, staring at the fountain in the garden, the sculpture of the girl holding the urn. I watched the water pulsing from the concrete vessel.

Felixstowe Hospital and the events of my past had not escaped my mind. The past existed like a foreign object in my head. It niggled and irritated my brain. Its message was unrelenting – you're mad and bad, you're mad and bad, over and over. With each tablet I swallowed, the message was reinforced. The chemicals coursed through my veins. My mind tried to filter the stench of this infection. I was getting accustomed to my feelings of terror.

I went inside into the formal lounge room and I stared at the fish in the aquarium. If I acknowledge Doctor Jarvie and her attempts to heal my sick mind, then perhaps there is hope? I had to believe in something, in my illness because it had now become my identity. There was nothing else.

I was still holding on to the brochure that the doctor had given me. I opened it and read its contents.

Pine View community house is a live-in residence providing programmes and support for mental health consumers. It aims to develop strategies to create an improved quality of life for those suffering with a mental illness.

Programmes include life skills, domestic functioning with budgeting advice, financial awareness, cooking and options for housing. Recreational, social integration, personal growth and relaxation are also part of the programme schedule.

I looked at the comprehensive list of tools and techniques used in managing mental illness. It included cognitive behavioural therapy, improving self-esteem and confidence, anger and anxiety management, dealing with depression, understanding mood disorder.

I was already tired and anxious and depressed just at the thought of this endeavour. I read the last item: goal setting with personal and professional development. On the last page of the brochure it had the contact details: Pine View reintegration facility, Cockatoo Crescent, Williamstown.

I was not impressed with this description of rehabilitation or the idea of living with others suffering from a mental illness. *To be cooped up in a house with weird people – how can the doctor think I would like such a thing? I'm not ill. I'm not like them.*

I couldn't help feeling I had gone back in time, to the setting of the film *To Sir With Love*, a movie about a school teaching impoverished or delinquent students how to survive in society. The financial realities of buying groceries came to mind.

I went to bed that night thinking of mandatory treatment and the necessity of placing individuals in certain sectors of society. I was placed in a category of 'mental illness' and therefore I had to be rehabilitated. I was given the option, of course, not to participate. This was not a dictatorship in the legal sense, but it had fascist social tendencies.

The terror of social exclusion, exiled from being a respected citizen, is what caused my pain. I felt their treatment contradicted all laws of medicine to make a person well. I was in fear of the system and it was not a physical abuse I had undergone. I felt I was mentally inferior. Perhaps it was just as well mental illness was invisible. It gave me some hope. I did not have a tattoo to brand me. My scar was on the inside.

Perhaps if I had done something wrong or had committed a crime or hurt another person, then I would have understood the terms of punishment as it related to the current judicial system. But I had gone to a hospital asking for help. The realisation that the medical system had perpetuated and increased my suffering made my head spin. I knew it was going on in the world all the time. Lawsuits were happening continuously in regard to medical negligence. For me, this was not one incident, to have made a mistake. This was continual. I would be spending the rest of my days taking their medication accessing their respective rehabilitative systems, asking for their benevolent help.

Medicine's scientific 'theology' classified me as delusional. I was subjected to inhumane treatment to change this so called 'difference'. When I was forced to accept their definition, then in their mind my recovery was possible. Their treatments were aimed at restoring my sanity but they had already acknowledged it as 'sick'. How could they redeem my core self when they had already disposed of it?

I knew I would not wake up refreshed with a new hope for a different day. The induced rest with sleeping tablets was artificial. I felt I was only a body of chemicals, a soulless entity.

The next day I saw the cleaners working in the hospital. I saw them everyday. They would wash my room, clean the floor and shower. Dust the furniture, place new linen on the bed and supply towels. Even a fresh jug of water was placed on the desk.

Each day, the nursing staff wandered the hospital. They would listen to the complaints and problems of patients. I found out later that the price of my staying in such a hospital cost the private insurance company over two thousand dollars a week. It was a large price to pay just to be given respect.

This was not a place for those who were destitute. The cost of private hospital insurance was high. I thought people who had major problems dealing with life would be the financially bereft. After all, it cost money to live and if you didn't have any, you would suffer. To me, it was common sense to help those who lived in poverty, but who could get well in Felixstowe?

The government at least did try to help those less fortunate. Basically it was the taxpayer giving money to others who did not work. Perhaps it was because of a sense of guilt that the system wanted to give to the poor and disabled. The politicians' popularity would increase, especially if there was a large percentage of the population on welfare. 'Here, have this money because I want to be in power next year.'

Living on a pension was difficult. I needed support financially. I couldn't afford to live on my own, making sure I had enough money to pay bills, rent, grocery shopping. Trying to make ends meet would be too difficult. I would have to think of other ways of accessing money.

I contemplated my future. I wanted to leave the medical system but I didn't have the confidence or the courage to walk away. I had to figure out a sensible approach, my reasons for treatment and how it would benefit me.

I had tried before participating in groups. The pottery didn't help and my painting had gone down the drain. When I did venture into the craft room, I tried to paint a landscape from my mind but it looked more like a collage of a burst water drain. The personal growth groups I had attended in the city, was like another form of sadistic therapy. I couldn't even sit in a room with other people, my fears were so intense. When I returned to my university studies, the lecturer noted that my ideas were novel. I lost interest in studying social sciences partly due to my social anxieties. I needed help but did not know how to remedy the situation.

I went to the red phones. I had some change in my pocket and placed a fifty-cent coin into the slot. I rang my mother.

'Mum, the doctor said I should go into a home. I don't believe it. How could she say that? She can't do that, can she?'

'I don't think she would want that. You must have misunderstood, Gardenia.'

'The doctor said that you needed a rest and if I went away it would be good for both of us. You'd have time out from me,' I said.

'I see.'

'As if it's entirely my fault!'

'I don't think she meant any harm, Gardenia. Did she say where this place was?'

'It's a community house in Williamstown. I read the brochure. I'd be living with other people with a mental illness. The doctor said that you'd get help from government services, like shopping, cleaning, that sort of thing.'

'I see.'

'You don't think it's a good idea, do you?'

'I think you should do what you want to do, Gardenia. It's your life and I'm still healthy. We can work it out. Come home, Gardenia.'

'I can learn self-help techniques from books without having to immerse myself in the mental health system. I can go to personal growth groups outside of a hospital situation. There are many things that I can do to improve myself.'

'Take it one step at a time, Gardenia.'

That's all you can do, really.

I felt that I had come through the worst. I had traversed the world of the shadows. Lived in a lost land and watched unspeakable horrors. I did not want to go on this journey, but I was forced to face the human condition. My own desperate pleas for help were lost in a system that could not act otherwise.

The world was a conundrum, a mystery that I could not understand. My intent to get better was genuine and I hoped one day to understand the cause of my affliction. I knew I could not just blame the mental health system. There was another reason for my illness, but to contemplate the possibilities; to ponder the unknown was frightening. Yet I had to face life and each new day was another beginning.

Appendix

Medications and side effects

Medications

The majority of Gardenia Baxter's medications were taken at Felixstowe Hospital and as an outpatient for the successive seven years.

Antipsychotics were prescribed for a psychotic thought disorder. Gardenia was later diagnosed with schizo-affective disorder.

Antipsychotics

Chlorpromazine
Thioridazine
Trifluoperazine
Haloperidol
Fluphenazine
Risperidone
Perphenazine

Gardenia was also diagnosed with depression and a generalised anxiety disorder.

Antidepressants

Imipramine
Dothiepin
Fluoxetine
Sertraline
Venlafaxine

Gardenia was also diagnosed with a bipolar-type disorder.

Mood stabilisers and anticonvulsants

Lithium
Sodium valproate
Carbamazepine
Lamotrigine

Gardenia also suffered with insomnia, anxiety and agitation.

Benzodiazepines

Lorazepam
Clonazepam
Diazepam
Alprazolam
Oxazepam

Gardenia was treated for side effects of medication.

Anticholinergics

Benzatropine
Orphenadrine

Side effects

Gardenia Baxter's list of unwanted side affects related to her psychiatric medication. There are greater degrees of discomfort attributable to some medications than others. Gardenia had signs of tardive dyskinesia and Parkinsonism symptoms.

Dilation of pupils – a significant and obvious sign of being over-medicated
Drowsiness, fatigue
Poor memory
Slowed intellectual functioning
Headache
Difficulty in speech
Disturbed concentration
Inability to sleep
Loss of appetite
Nausea
Vomiting
Mask-like face
Decreased frequency of blinking
Inability to move eyes
Blurred vision
Muscle spasms of face
Difficulty in swallowing
Disorientation
Restlessness or need to keep moving
Shuffling walk; stiffness of arms or legs
Trembling and shaking of hands and fingers
Involuntary choreathetotic movements
Slow movements
Walking stiffly without swinging the arms
Stooped posture
Loss of balance and control
Lack or loss of coordination
Dizziness
Seizures
Weight gain
Diabetes
Swelling of ankles
Swollen lips
Dryness of mouth
Nasal stuffiness
Increased perspiration
Constipation
Acne
Fluid retention
Difficulty in urinating
Numbness
Sensitivity to light
Aggression
Anger
Hostility
Irritability
Socially inappropriate behaviour – for example, disrobing in public
Breast enlargement
Changes in menstrual period
Elevated prolactin, which suppresses menstruation

www.ingramcontent.com/pod-product-compliance
Lightning Source LLC
Chambersburg PA
CBHW021829020426
42334CB00014B/544